Complementary and Alternative Medicine

AN ILLUSTRATED COLOUR TEXT

For Elsevier Churchill Livingstone

Commissioning Editor: Ellen Green
Development Editor: Helen Leng
Project Manager: Frances Affleck
Designer: Erik Bigland
Illustrator: Bruce Hogarth
Cartoons: David Banks

Complementary and Alternative Medicine

AN ILLUSTRATED COLOUR TEXT

Edited by

Allan D Cumming BSc(Hons) MBChB MD FRCP(E)
Professor of Medical Education and Director of Undergraduate Learning and Teaching
Honorary Consultant Physician
College of Medicine and Veterinary Medicine
University of Edinburgh, UK

Karen R Simpson BA(Hons) RN RNT
Fellow in Medical Education
College of Medicine and Veterinary Medicine
University of Edinburgh, UK

David Brown MBChB, DRCOG
General Practitioner
Murrayfield Medical Centre
Edinburgh, UK
Honorary Clinical Tutor
University of Edinburgh, UK

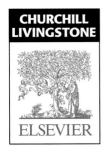

EDINBURGH   LONDON   NEW YORK   OXFORD   PHILADELPHIA   ST LOUIS   SYDNEY   TORONTO   2007

CHURCHILL LIVINGSTONE
ELSEVIER

First published 2007

ISBN 10: 0443073740
ISBN 13: 978-0-443-07374-8

British Library Cataloguing in Publication Data
A catalogue record for this book is available from the British Library

Library of Congress Cataloging in Publication Data
A catalog record for this book is available from the Library of Congress

---

Notice

Neither the publisher nor the authors assume any responsibility for any loss or injury and/or damage to persons or property arising out of or related to any use of the material contained in this book. It is the responsibility of the treating practitioner, relying on independent expertise and knowledge of the patient, to determine the best treatment and method of application for the patient.

The Publisher

---

your source for books, journals and multimedia in the health sciences
www.elsevierhealth.com

Working together to grow libraries in developing countries

www.elsevier.com | www.bookaid.org | www.sabre.org

ELSEVIER | BOOK AID International | Sabre Foundation

The Publisher's policy is to use **paper manufactured from sustainable forests**

Printed in China

Contributors

Bryan Allan RGN RSCN
Clinical Communication Skills Deputy
  Theme Head
Coordinator Simulated Patient Programme
College of Medicine and Veterinary
  Medicine
University of Edinburgh, UK

Kirsty J Boyd MBChB FRCP
Honorary Clinical Senior Lecturer
Clinical Communication Skills Theme
  Head
Community Health Sciences
General Practice Section
University of Edinburgh, UK

David Brown MBChB DRCOG
General Practitioner
Murrayfield Medical Centre, Edinburgh
Honorary Clinical Tutor
University of Edinburgh, UK

James P M Campbell MD FLCOM
  DM-Smed MSc
Consultant in Musculoskeletal Medicine
Royal Infirmary of Edinburgh
Edinburgh, UK

Allan D Cumming BSc(Hons)
  MBChB MD FRCP(E)
Professor of Medical Education and
  Director of Undergraduate Learning
  and Teaching
Honorary Consultant Physician
College of Medicine and Veterinary
  Medicine
University of Edinburgh, UK

Alastair Dobbin MB BS DipClinHyp
General Practitioner
Edinburgh, UK

Marshall F Dozier MA PdDipLIS
Deputy Theme Head for Evidence Based
  Medicine
Liaison Librarian for Medicine
University of Edinburgh, UK

Marie Fallon MBChB FRCP(G)
  FRCP(E) MRCGP DCH DRCOG
St Columba's Hospice Chair in Palliative
  Medicine
Edinburgh Cancer Centre
Edinburgh, UK

Scott A Murray MBChB MD FRCGP
  FRCP(E) DRCOG DCH
St Columba's Hospice Chair in Primary
  Palliative Care
Division of Community Health Sciences
College of Medicine and Veterinary
  Medicine
University of Edinburgh, UK

Mike Porter BA MPhil
Senior Lecturer
General Practice Section
Division of Community Health Sciences
College of Medicine and Veterinary
  Medicine
University of Edinburgh, UK

Margaret R Ritchie BSc(Hons) BEd
  PhD
Teaching and Research Fellow
Cancer Biology Group
Bute Medical School
University of St Andrews
St Andrews, UK

Michael T Ross BSc(Hons) MBChB
  DRCOG MRCGP
Clinical Lecturer in General Practice
Fellow in Medical Education
College of Medicine and Veterinary
  Medicine
University of Edinburgh, UK

Karen R Simpson BA(Hons) RN RNT
Fellow in Medical Education
College of Medicine and Veterinary
  Medicine
University of Edinburgh, UK

Janet Skinner MBChB FRCS(E)
  MMed ED FFAEM
Specialist Registrar
Emergency Medicine
Royal Infirmary of Edinburgh
Edinburgh, UK

Thomas E Whitmarsh MA FRCP
  FFHom
Consultant Physician
Glasgow Homeopathic Hospital
Glasgow, UK

Preface

As will be emphasised and documented later in this book, complementary and alternative medicine (CAM) is a growth industry. There are many reasons for the increasing popularity of CAM, and these will be discussed later in the book. However, the days when medical schools and other healthcare schools could afford to ignore the existence of CAM and dismiss it as 'superstitious medieval nonsense' are long gone. Five hundred years ago, universities and medical schools were appointed to be the custodians and providers of orthodox medical knowledge. As scientific knowledge has advanced our understanding of disease processes, leading to new approaches to diagnosis and treatment based on firm scientific principles, it is not too surprising that a divergence has occurred between CAM and orthodox medicine and that barriers have developed. More recently the adoption of evidence-based medicine as a rubric for most medical situations has widened the gap.

Education is at the heart of this; indeed one definition of CAM is anything that is not taught at medical school. Whatever one's view of the nature, efficacy, and validity of individual CAM therapies, it is clearly undesirable for conventional practitioners to be in ignorance of treatments which are being used by more than half of their patients. That is one reason why all medical schools, at least in the UK, now include some exposure to and familiarisation with complementary and alternative medicine within their undergraduate curricula. Within that broad statement there lies a wide variety of practice, ranging from full-blown formal courses and linked assessments, to optional attachments which meet the needs of particular students with interests in this area. Few if any medical schools require students to develop practical expertise in the techniques of CAM, although this is often possible within student-selected components for the motivated student. The Education Committee of the General Medical Council, who inspect and accredit all medical schools in the UK, have driven this process actively. Their guidance in 'Tomorrow's Doctors' on undergraduate medical education includes the statement that:

> …students must be aware that many patients are interested in and choose to use a range of alternative and complementary therapies. Graduates must be aware of the existence and range of such therapies, why some patients use them, and how these might affect other types of treatment that patients are receiving. (GMC 2002)

The high prevalence of CAM use means that CAM is an issue which permeates all aspects of students' experiences while at medical school. Many of the patients whom they meet during the training will be using CAM. Thus at any point in their course, they may be required to think about, write about and reflect on issues related to complementary medicine. The aim of this short text is to provide the information which all healthcare students might need in these situations. The text covers various general aspects of CAM, followed by brief summary details of the more common forms of CAM therapy. Particular attention has been given to issues such as communication and consultation, ethics and legal responsibilities, which often form important vertical themes in medical curricula.

The book has been prepared and edited by a team of medical professionals (a hospital doctor, a general practitioner and a registered nurse) all of whom have a close interest in complementary medicine and, in particular, in teaching and learning in this area. All are closely involved in teaching medical students and in formulating curriculum learning objectives and assessments. The contributors are from a range of backgrounds, including orthodox and complementary practitioners. We believe that the book represents a balanced attempt to support the integration of CAM into medical and other healthcare-related curricula. It also provides directions to information sources to facilitate further study in particular areas.

Both conventional and complementary medicine have the patient's well-being as their primary concern. From that standpoint, there can be no argument for isolationist, defensive attitudes which leave patients uncertain and confused. There is every incentive to develop improved mutual understanding and enhanced inter-professional communication and cooperation. Enhanced education is an important step along the way.

AC, KS, DB

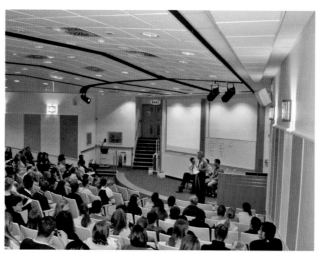

Edinburgh University medical students. (Photograph courtesy of University of Edinburgh.)

Contents

Introduction to complementary and alternative medicine and overview

What is complementary and alternative medicine?

Allan D. Cumming

Many terms are used when referring to different complementary and alternative treatments (Table 1). However, as most forms of treatment can be used in a variety of ways, the term complementary and alternative medicine (CAM) tends to be used generically in the United Kingdom. CAM can be defined as a group of medical and healthcare systems, practices and products that are not considered to be part of conventional medicine (Fig. 1). A more lengthy definition used by the Cochrane Collaboration is:

> a broad domain of healing resources that encompasses all health systems, modalities and practices and their accompanying theories and beliefs, other than those intrinsic to the politically dominant health systems of a particular society or culture in a given historical period. (Zollman & Vickers 1999d)

The British Medical Association (BMA) uses the definition:

> those forms of treatment which are not widely used by the conventional health care professions, and the skills of which are not taught as part of the undergraduate curriculum of conventional medical and paramedical health care courses. (BMA 1993)

This definition emphasises the importance of education and training in maintaining the traditional boundaries between CAM and conventional medicine (Berman 2001). This is very much the theme of this book, and will be explored further.

In each of these three cases the definition is essentially one of exclusion – conventional medicine is clearly defined and recognised, anything outside those boundaries is complementary and alternative medicine. Those boundaries are, however, becoming less distinct. More and more health centres, community treatment centres, and hospital units offer an integrated package of treatment modalities, where patients may experience conventional and CAM therapy, often at the same visit, or even from the same practitioner (Dobson 2003). CAM is moving forward in areas such as

professional regulation and evidence base that have separated it from mainstream medicine. How far this integration will eventually proceed remains to be seen. Nevertheless, it is clear that neither constituency can afford to remain ignorant of the other, and that mutual understanding and collaboration are in the best interests of patient care (Rees & Weil 2001).

These definitions cover an enormous and ever-changing range of CAM activities, from well-established physical therapies such as osteopathy to spiritual measures such as prayer specifically for health. Some of the more commonly used or accepted CAM therapies are familiar to healthcare professionals. However, as the use of CAM becomes more popular within the Western world the list is ever increasing; therefore with the vast number of CAM therapies available it is helpful to categorise them to enable doctors and others to place each therapy, both new and old, in context with others.

Categorising complementary and alternative medicine

There are a variety of ways to categorise CAM therapies. Pietroni (1991) devised one of the first classifications which

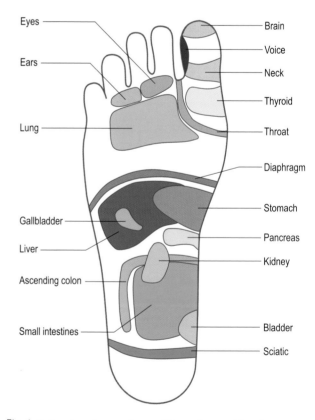

Fig. 1 **Reflexology is one of several therapies considered as complementary and alternative medicine which are not considered conventional medicine.**

Table 1 **Frequently used terms**	
Complementary medicine	Non-conventional treatments used along with conventional medicine, e.g. acupuncture to reduce pain
Alternative medicine	Non-conventional treatments used in place of conventional medicine, e.g. using reflexology instead of anti-inflammatory drugs for arthritis
Integrative medicine	When conventional therapy is combined with one or more complementary therapies for which there is evidence of efficacy and safety
Natural medicine	Any non-conventional medicine
Holistic medicine	Focuses on the whole person, their lifestyle, environment, diet, and their mental, emotional and spiritual health, as well as their physical complaints. CAM proponents suggest that, unlike most of conventional medicine, its therapies are holistic

was used by the British Medical Association in their report in 1993. However, in 2000 in the United Kingdom, the House of Lords Select Committee on Science and Technology report derived a classification with three groups, which is used more frequently (Table 2).

In the United States, the classification system of the National Center for Complementary and Alternative Medicine (NCCAM) is used. Each classification gives a generic description of the theory or premise on which the CAM therapies placed within each group are based (Table 3).

Safety

Not all complementary and alternative therapies are safe (Burton 2003). Some are toxic in their own right, e.g. dietary supplements containing ephedrine alkaloids which have been banned in the US. Others are harmful used in combination with other CAM or conventional treatment, e.g. garlic supplements interfering with the action of anti-HIV

chemotherapy. There is also potential for harm through patients using CAM in preference to conventional medicine for symptoms of serious or life-threatening medical conditions.

Evidence

Practitioners and advocates of CAM are often challenged to justify these treatments through independent, well-conducted, randomised controlled clinical trials (RCTs). In some cases this is difficult – the placebo arm of a double-blind trial of acupuncture, for example. However, the literature in this area is growing rapidly. At present a minority of CAM therapies are supported by evidence that would be acceptable for conventional medicine (UK BEAM 2004a, 2004b, Harlow et al 2004). Where evidence does exist, it is often limited to a small subset of the clinical conditions for which the treatment is used, or a specific clinical context (Vas et al 2004). It has been argued that different types and standards of evidence, focusing on patient satisfaction and subjective benefit rather than measurable clinical outcomes, should be considered in the case of CAM (see below). The doctor's perspective on CAM, including the efficacy, safety and evidence issues surrounding CAM, must be understood by healthcare professionals, users of CAM and CAM practitioners.

Incidental or placebo effects

The effects of any medical intervention can be considered as characteristic (specific) and incidental (placebo, non-specific) elements. In the testing of new drugs in conventional medicine, the characteristic effects are normally isolated by the use of a dummy (placebo) preparation in a proportion of subjects who are selected from the study cohort at random. Each subject, and the researcher, would normally be unaware of whether the active or dummy preparation is being administered until after the observations have been completed (the double-blind, placebo-controlled randomised clinical trial, Fig. 3). The characteristic effects of the drug are identified by comparing the outcomes in those receiving the active drug with the outcomes in those receiving the dummy preparation (Mason et al 2002).

Such study designs are used because effects, both positive and negative, are observed with any medical intervention, even where the drug or substance being administered is known to be inert. This is often known as the placebo effect. Incidental factors have been shown to affect outcome – for example, the extent to which the patient believes in the therapy, the expectations of the patient from the consultation, the general approach of the practitioner, and the setting in which the treatment is delivered. In order to justify the costs of manufacturing and dispensing active drugs, it must be shown that they are superior to dummy preparations and that this superiority is related to characteristic (specific) factors rather than incidental factors.

However, in most CAM therapies, it is much less straightforward to separate out the characteristic and incidental effects (Paterson & Dieppe 2005). For example, in conventional RCTs, the assumption is made that a diagnosis of the condition being treated has been made before the trial intervention begins, that the treatment is carried out for a known condition, and the treatment is not 'contaminated' by the process of diagnosis. However, in acupuncture, the

Table 2 **House of Lords Select Committee's CAM taxonomy (House of Lords 2000)**	
Group 1	Most established forms of CAM in the Western world that have a particular form of diagnostic method and are the most advanced in terms of regulated practice, and in general, are the strongest in terms of evidence for efficacy. Often referred to as the 'big five' therapies
Therapies	Osteopathy, chiropractic, acupuncture, herbal medicine and homeopathy
Group 2	Therapies that are normally used to complement conventional medicine, and do not claim to make diagnoses
Therapies	Aromatherapy, Alexander technique, body work therapies such as massage, counselling, stress therapy; hypnotherapy; reflexology, shiatsu, meditation and healing
Group 3	Therapies that offer diagnostic as well as therapeutic services. They involve a philosophy which does not relate to conventional medical science, and through which various mechanisms of disease causation and management are put forward. They split into two subgroups (3a and 3b)
Group 3a therapies	Includes established, traditional systems of healthcare such as Ayurvedic medicine and traditional Chinese medicine
Group 3b therapies	Includes a number of disciplines which lack an evidence base: crystal therapy, iridology, radionics, dowsing and kinesiology

Table 3 **NCCAM classification system for CAM therapies (NCCAM 2004)**	
Alternative medical systems	Therapies that have their own constructs of theory and practice, often based on ancient historical beliefs
Therapies	Homeopathy, naturopathy, traditional Chinese medicine, and Ayurveda
Mind–body interactions	Therapies relying on the mind's capacity to influence physical function
Therapies	Hypnosis, meditation, prayer, mental healing, music therapy and dance
Biologically based	Therapies involving the use or regulation of an extraneous agent or preparation
Therapies	Herbal medicine, dietary supplementation, and nutritional medicine
Manipulative and body-based	Therapies based on manipulation or movement of parts of the body
Therapies	Osteopathy, chiropractic, reflexology, and massage, which is often combined with aromatherapy
Energy based	Therapies involving use of energy fields
Therapies	Gi gong, reiki, and therapeutic touch

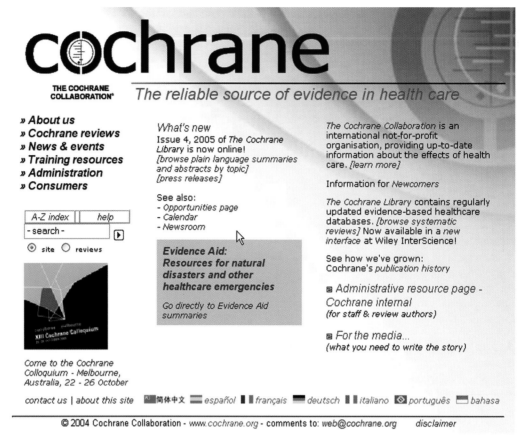

Fig. 2 **Opening web page of the Cochrane Collaboration site.** (Reproduced with permission of The Cochrane Collaboration.)

diagnosis (expressed in terms of Chinese medicine) is made in an emergent fashion during a course of treatment. This progressive process of diagnosis is specific to Chinese medicine, and is therefore associated with a characteristic rather than an incidental effect.

It is also assumed that incidental factors are essentially generic, and not linked to any particular intervention. However, it is clear that for many CAM therapies, factors such as talking and listening to the patient are integral to the treatment process, and cannot be considered as incidental. The classic placebo-controlled RCT design assumes that characteristic effects and incidental effects are simply additive, and that one class of effect can be easily subtracted from the other in an arithmetic fashion. It has been argued, however, that for complex interventions such as most CAM therapies, this is not appropriate. The use of placebo- or sham-controlled trial designs in such a context will not detect the whole characteristic effect and may therefore generate false-negative results. Other approaches, such as randomised pragmatic designs and randomised cluster designs, have been recommended (Paterson & Dieppe 2005).

Regulation of CAM

The 'big five' CAM therapies have their own professional regulatory frameworks in place, and others are following suit (Mills 2001a). Nevertheless, for many CAM therapies, there is no established structure of training, certification and accreditation, and practice is effectively open to all. This often contrasts with the demanding entry qualifications, training and lifelong continuous professional development that pertains to conventional medicine (see Section 2).

Communication

In the UK, relationships between CAM and conventional medicine, at institutional and individual levels, are not always harmonious. There is not a tradition of open communication and collaboration over the care of individual patients. A key aspect of the education and training of practitioners of both types must be to emphasise the need

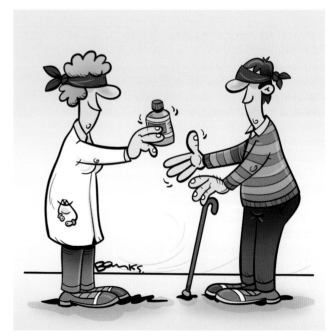

Fig. 3 **A double-blind placebo-controlled clinical trial for CAM therapies.**

to share relevant information in the best interests of patients. The section on communication highlights the key aspects required to maintain good communication of practitioner to practitioner and patient to practitioner (see Section 5).

Summary

CAM is popular and increasingly is being integrated with conventional medicine. CAM is being categorised, described, and regulated more than before, although many important issues remain. The extent to which CAM should be subjected to the same demands for evidence of efficacy as conventional treatments, and the feasibility of doing so, is a key question.

Education and training for both CAM and conventional practitioners is crucial to the future of well-coordinated patient care.

Sources of further information

- House of Lords Select Committee Science and Technology 2000 Complementary and alternative medicine, 6th report. Online. Available: http://www.parliament.the-stationery-office.co.uk/pa/ld199900/ldselect/ldsctech/123/12301.htm
- National Center for Complementary and Alternative Medicine. Established by the US Congress in 1998. Online. Available: http://nccam.nih.gov

Learning about CAM: reasons, recommendations and strategies

Allan D. Cumming

Statutory recommendations

The UK General Medical Council, in their report 'Tomorrow's Doctors', stated that medical students must be:

> aware that many patients are interested in and choose to use a range of alternative and complementary therapies. Graduates must be aware of the existence and range of such therapies, why some patients use them, and how these might affect other types of treatment that patients are receiving. (GMC 2002)

In their report on an informal visit to the University of Edinburgh Medical School in 2000, the GMC Education Committee suggested that more teaching about CAM should be introduced to the undergraduate curriculum, so that graduates would be 'as informed about complementary medicine as their future patients' (GMC 2000). This recommendation has been criticised because curriculum planners do not necessarily know how informed future patients will be, especially about specific forms of CAM.

The House of Lords Select Committee on Science and Technology, in their report on CAM, stated:

> We recommend that familiarization should prepare medical students for dealing with patients who are either accessing CAM or have an interest in doing so. This familiarization should cover the potential uses of CAM, the procedures involved, their potential benefits and their main weaknesses and dangers. We recommend that every medical school ensures that all their medical undergraduates are exposed to a level of CAM familiarization that makes them aware of the choices their patients might make. (Mills 2001a)

It is clear that UK government and statutory bodies are exerting considerable pressure on medical schools to incorporate additional content related to CAM into their curricula. Most UK medical schools, but not all, have allowed interested students the opportunity to study CAM as a 'student-selected component' or option, and in the core curriculum, have taught about the existence of CAM in relation to public health and illness behaviour. However, to answer the stipulations of the GMC and the House of Lords requires most schools to considerably alter their curriculum content and the general approach to CAM.

Reasons for recommendations

There are numerous reasons why statutory bodies are recommending more CAM in medical curricula. These include:

- increasing popularity of CAM and prevalence of CAM use in the Western world
- increasing public knowledge and understanding about CAM
- increasing public expectation that conventional practitioners will be familiar with CAM and have understanding of it
- a belief that conventional medical practice can be informed and enhanced through interactions with the field of CAM
- a belief that in many circumstances, integrated healthcare may be better than either type of care alone, and may be in the best interests of many patients
- the perception that educational patterns and traditions are a major barrier to the growth of integrated care.

Popularity and growing use of CAM

In Western society, the use and provision of CAM is extensive and growing (Fig. 4). A telephone survey in 1999 suggested that 20% of adults in the UK had used some form of CAM in the previous 12 months (Ernst 2000). The average amount spent was £14 per month, suggesting an annual spend on CAM in the UK of around £1.6 billion. It has been estimated that spending on CAM in the UK is increasing by 50% every 5 years (Thomas et al 2001). In 2002 in the United States, at any one time 36% of the population were using some form of CAM. If prayer for health reasons was included, this rose to 62% (NCCAM).

The most common medical conditions involved were back, neck, head or joint pain, upper respiratory tract infections, anxiety or depression, gastrointestinal symptoms, and sleep disturbance. As long ago as 1997, the number of visits to CAM practitioners in the US was 629 million (Eisenberg et al 1998). This exceeded visits to all primary care medical practitioners. It is estimated that in the US and Europe, the amount paid to CAM practitioners comfortably exceeds fees for physician services and hospitalisation for conventional medicine. A study in 2000 suggested that there were approximately 50 000 CAM practitioners in the UK, of whom about 10 000 were statutorily registered (Mills & Budd 2000). Clearly, this popularity of CAM is relevant for future medical practitioners, and must have significance for the practice of conventional medicine. By seeking the reasons which underlie the popularity, much may be learned about the doctor–patient relationship, definitions of health, patterns of illness behaviour, patient perspectives, and other key aspects of healthcare (Table 4).

It is clear that students of conventional medicine must be aware of the existence of CAM and be familiar with at least the more common forms of therapy. However, this is not just related to their ability to deal with these issues when interacting with patients. It also relates to a deeper understanding of how medicine works and the factors that determine the success or failure of therapeutic processes.

Integrating CAM into medical curricula

There is an extensive literature on how CAM can be integrated into conventional medical curricula. The most prevalent

Table 4 **Learning points from widespread CAM usage**
■ The importance of personal experience in determining health and illness behaviour and underlying attitudes
■ The ways in which patients' beliefs about health and medicine influence their interactions with healthcare systems and individual therapists
■ The importance which patients attach to the safety of any treatment
■ The willingness of some patients to gamble in relation to health
■ The distrust and fear of conventional medicine which exists in society, and the factors which underlie it; potential strategies to reverse it
■ The reluctance of some patients to declare their illness, and conversely, the desire of other patients to adopt an illness role
■ The importance of patient choice in healthcare provision
■ The importance of unhurried, comprehensible, patient-centred communication as part of a consultation
■ Financial issues as determinants of patient behaviour
■ Cultural, ethnic and societal issues as determinants of patient behaviour
■ The importance of communication, understanding and mutual respect between different healthcare disciplines
■ The importance of teamwork in healthcare

approach is to offer students 'elective' or optional attachments to CAM practices and practitioners. However, many medical schools have noted that demand for such experience among students is low and the level of uptake of opportunities is disappointing (Owen & Lewith 2001). Clearly this reflects current attitudes among students of conventional medicine. In order to break this cycle, it is necessary that CAM also be integrated in the core curriculum of medical schools (Fig. 5).

Strategies to integrate CAM into medical schools

Strategy I: Be as informed as their future patients
This strategy enables students to familiarise themselves with a range of complementary therapies, and allows them to be aware of the choices that their patients might make, and their reasons for making them.

Strategy II: Evidence and efficacy
This strategy enables students to demonstrate their ability to appraise complementary therapies in terms of evidence base, concentrating on those therapies with evidence for efficacy, but also understanding the different types of evidence that there are.

Strategy III: Illness behaviour and psychological aspects
This approach ensures that students are able to explain the reasons why patients seek complementary therapies, including the importance of the therapeutic consultation, communication skills and issues of compliance.

Strategy IV: Understand the 'big five' therapies
This tactic ensures that students are able to demonstrate a broad understanding of the five main complementary therapies that have professional regulatory systems in place. This includes knowledge of evidence base, indications and interactions.

Clearly these strategies are not mutually exclusive, although the pressure to include content in medical curricula means that in most cases a degree of selectivity is necessary.

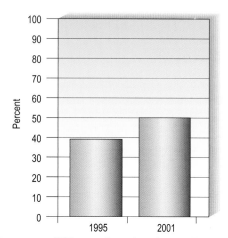

Fig. 4 **Percentage of UK general practices that provide CAM services.** (Thomas et al 2001.)

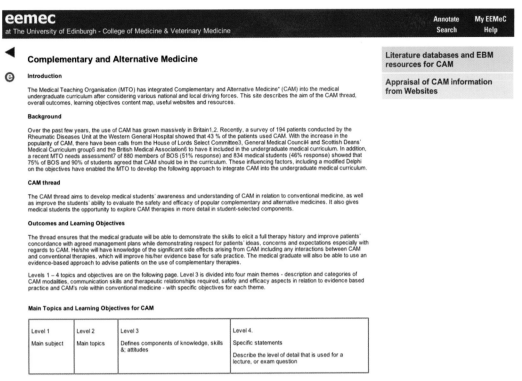

Fig. 5 **Edinburgh Electronic Medical Curriculum (EEMeC) with CAM page.** (Courtesy of University of Edinburgh.)

Learning outcomes for healthcare students

A set of CAM learning outcomes for healthcare students that covers the three domains (knowledge, skills and attitudes) can help students to understand what it is they need to learn.

The following set of learning outcomes/competences has been developed by the University of Edinburgh medical school, and is an example of this type of outcome-based approach.

By the end of their undergraduate course, students should be able to demonstrate the following:

Knowledge
1. Discuss the reasons why patients choose to use complementary treatments or to consult with an alternative practitioner.
2. Describe the importance of psychological, spiritual and social issues in the management of patients.
3. Describe how different members of the expanded healthcare team, including complementary therapists, can play important roles in patient management.
4. Describe the importance of osteopathy and chiropractic in managing musculoskeletal disorders, such as back pain, including the efficacy of these therapies.
5. Discuss the use of complementary therapies, particularly acupuncture in the management of chronic pain.
6. Explain the potential seriousness of interactions that can occur between complementary therapies and conventional therapies including accessing accurate information about these interactions.
7. Describe the use of herbal medicines in psychiatry, including the evidence base.
8. Discuss the growing use of homeopathic medications in many medical conditions.

9. Describe how complementary medicine fits with, and relates to, conventional medicine.
10. Discuss the growing use of complementary therapies by Western populations.
11. Discuss the use of complementary therapies within healthcare systems outside the Western world.

Skills
1. Discuss therapeutic choices with patients, including complementary therapies (Fig. 6).
2. Elicit a history of complementary therapy use during a patient consultation, including the patient's reasons for using them.
3. Critically appraise the evidence in support of efficacy of complementary therapies.

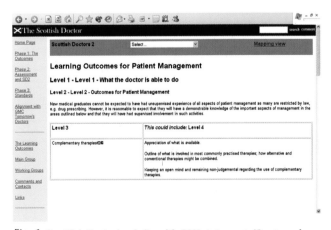

Fig. 6 **'Scottish Doctor' website with CAM statement.** (Courtesy of Scottish Deans Medical Curriculum group.)

Attitudes

1. Appreciate the individuality of patients and that each patient has the right to be involved in decision-making about their treatment.
2. Learn from patients, all members of the primary healthcare team and other resources in the community.
3. Appreciate the importance of clear communication between different individuals involved in patient care.
4. Recognise the importance of the consultation with the complementary therapist, including the 'therapeutic touch'.
5. Maintain an open mind about alternative approaches to patient care.
6. Appreciate that not all patients will disclose their use of complementary therapies to a conventional practitioner, and reasons why this may be.
7. Respect the rights of patients to choose different forms of therapy or to attend a range of practitioners.

Examples of approaches to CAM teaching

1. A detailed attitudinal survey and needs analysis in the University of Edinburgh Medical School in 2002 confirmed that both staff and students generally support the integration of CAM into the undergraduate medical curriculum, but with concerns among both groups about efficacy, validity and regulation. A modified-Delphi process suggested that CAM teaching should provide students with a broad overall familiarisation with CAM, but with an emphasis throughout on critically evaluating evidence for efficacy. An integrated core course running through all years of the curriculum was preferred, using a variety of teaching methods, including an experiential component for all students.
2. Review of the issues surrounding the introduction of CAM teaching to medical schools, based on experience in the University of Maryland (Berman 2001).
3. Description of CAM teaching at undergraduate medical school (Owen et al 2001).
4. A comparative analysis of attitudes toward CAM among medical, nursing, and pharmacy faculty and students (Kreitzer et al 2002).

Ethics, law and professional issues

Ethics

Allan D. Cumming

The concept that all medical treatment should be delivered according to an ethical code dates back to ancient times (e.g. the Hippocratic Oath). In the case of conventional medicine, there is a long-established academic discipline of medical ethics. In the UK, the Institute of Medical Ethics has established a professional journal, the *Journal of Medical Ethics* (http://jme.bmjjournals.com), and has conducted important reviews of medical ethics education and practice. There is also a well-established network in the UK related specifically to clinical medical ethics (http://www.ethics-network.org.uk/index.htm). Medical disasters such as the activities of Dr Harold Shipman have increased the degree of ethical scrutiny to which conventional medicine is exposed. The UK General Medical Council have issued detailed guidance about the duties of a doctor, the ethical standards to which doctors should adhere in their practice, and how doctors should be educated and trained in this regard (http://www.gmc-uk.org/guidance/library/duties_of_a_doctor.asp; http://www.gmc-uk.org/guidance/good_medical_practice/index.asp; http://www.gmc-uk.org/education/index.asp).

Ethical issues are also clearly relevant to the practice of complementary and alternative medicine. Many of the CAM professional associations publish an ethical code of conduct (Table 5). Many also help to educate their members with regard to ethical principles and practice, and administer a system to deal with ethical issues when necessary. However, overall, the ethical framework within which CAM is practised, at least in the UK, is less well developed, standardised and defined than for conventional medicine. This has led to considerable attention being given to ethical practice as a general principle which should underlie both CAM and conventional medicine (Stone & Matthews 1996).

For example, a key medical ethical principle, which also impinges on legal issues, is that of confidentiality. This is particularly problematic in the case of a patient who is receiving treatment from both a conventional and an alternative practitioner. Many CAM therapies place particular emphasis on communication with the patient and elucidation of underlying personal or social difficulties. It is possible that a CAM practitioner may uncover information of undoubted importance for the patient's conventional medical care. The patient may or may not be happy for this information to be passed on. Here the principles of confidentiality and autonomy are important. Each case would need to be subjected to a process of ethical analysis to decide on the best course of action. In general, it seems likely that if the information was highly significant, to a degree that secrecy might lead to harm to the patient, the CAM practitioner would have an ethical, and potentially a legal, obligation to communicate with the conventional practitioner, and would be required to do their utmost to persuade the patient to agree to this. The converse would also apply, so that if the conventional practitioner became aware of a potential conflict between the two therapies or other important relevant information, it would incumbent on him to inform the CAM practitioner (British Medical Association 1993).

Another fundamental ethical principle is that of informed consent. Practices in this respect vary, so that, for example, a patient would always be required to sign a formal consent form before undergoing a surgical operation, but not normally before starting a course of antibiotics. However, it is generally expected that all patients undergoing any treatment are fully informed as to the nature of the proposed treatment, are made aware of the risks and possible side effects, and – where appropriate – have signed documentation to that effect prior to starting treatment. Although direct evidence is lacking, it seems likely that this may not always be the case in relation to CAM therapies. It can be argued that this is less relevant because most CAM therapies are either completely safe, or comparatively safe, in comparison to conventional treatments. The principle of *therapeutic privilege*, where it is viewed as kinder to the patient not to explain possible adverse effects, may be invoked. The assumption may also be made that where the patient chooses to consult a practitioner and to pay him a fee, consent is implied. Nevertheless, the principle of informed consent is fundamental to medical practice. Integrated healthcare may place greater requirements on CAM therapists in this respect.

Legal aspects of health care delivery

In the UK, both conventional medicine and CAM are subject to a generic, extensive and complex legal framework which applies to the delivery of all healthcare services. The most important is probably the Medicines Act of 1968 and subsequent amendments and additions (http://www.opsi.gov.uk/si/si1989/Uksi_19890192_en_1.htm) which regulate the quality and proven safety of drugs and substances used in medical treatments. Some forms of CAM remedies, such as herbal medicine preparations and certain products classed as nutritional supplements, have been exempted from the requirements of the Act, although this is under review.

The framework also includes laws about notification of disease (e.g. the Public Health Control of Disease Act 1984,

Table 5 **Ethical code of practice for osteopaths** (http://www.osteopathy.org.uk/)
An osteopath must:
■ put patients first
■ foster and maintain trust between themselves and their patients
■ listen to patients and respect their views
■ give patients the information they need and be sure that they understand
■ respect and protect confidential information
■ respect patients' autonomy and allow them choice
■ maintain and develop their professional knowledge and skills
■ practise within professional competence
■ never abuse their professional position
■ respect the skills of all other healthcare professionals and work in cooperation with them
■ respond promptly and constructively to criticism and complaints.

http://www.opsi.gov.uk/si/si1988/Uksi_19881546_en_1.htm)
and a large number of laws which regulate the standards
of the premises in which healthcare can be delivered.
All healthcare provision is also subject to laws relating
to use of and access to information (e.g. the Freedom of
Information Act 2000, http://www.opsi.gov.uk/acts/acts2000/
20000036.htm and the Data Protection Act 1998
http://www.opsi.gov.uk/acts/acts1998/19980029.htm).

The provision of either conventional medicine or CAM
is subject to civil law (law which concerns itself with rights
and obligations), which imposes a duty of care on any
practitioner towards their patient. A departure from this
duty of care may be found to be negligent. In conventional
medicine, negligence is often defined as failure to act in
accordance with the practice accepted as proper by a
responsible body of medical men skilled in that particular
area. This is often referred to as the Bolam test (Samanata &
Samanta 2003). However, defining such practice in relation
to most CAM therapies is more complicated than for
conventional medicine. For example, there is an important
issue concerning individualised treatment. In conventional
medicine, if two patients present to a practitioner with an
identical clinical picture, he is likely to treat them in an
identical fashion. This will often be determined by evidence-
based guidelines and protocols, previously agreed by a
consensus panel of experts in the field (e.g. the Scottish
Intercollegiate Guidelines Network, http://www.sign.ac.uk).
A significant departure from such guidelines, if detrimental
to the patient, may be found to be negligent. However it is
not unusual for two patients with the same condition to
be given completely different remedies by the same CAM
practitioner, based on a holistic assessment of their individual
needs. This makes the judgement of what is or is not
acceptable practice, and what might be negligent, much
more difficult (Ernst 2000).

Where care is provided on a private, fee-paying basis,
a contract is established between the practitioner and
their patient, and aspects of contract law apply
(http://www.sosig.ac.uk/roads/subject-listing/World-cat/
contractlaw.html is a useful link). Any healthcare practitioner
may also in some circumstances be liable under criminal
law. Relevant statutes include the Misrepresentation Act
1967, the Fair Trading Act 1983 and the Children's Act 1989.

Professional regulation and right to practise

The entitlement to practice conventional medicine is
governed by a long-established legal framework, embedded
in statutory law. For example, by UK and European law,
only graduates from a university can practise conventional
medicine. In the UK this dates back to the Medical Act of
1512, and the link between graduating from a university
and licensure to practise medicine has been maintained
in the UK and most other countries until now. Schools of
conventional medicine continue to be embedded in
universities, and the universities work closely with the state
and the professional regulatory bodies in relation to standards
and competences for new doctors. In contrast, although
graduate degree courses in CAM are increasingly prevalent,
there is no legal requirement for such qualifications in order
to practise CAM. This schism dates from the 16th century,
when the fees of registered graduate medical practitioners
were more than most people could afford. In 1542 the
Herbalists Charter was passed which stated that anyone
could legally practise herbal medicine. However, under the
law, charges had to be limited, and confined only to the cost
of the herbal preparation. To date, in the UK it is still the
case that in law, anyone can practise complementary and
alternative medicine, irrespective of their qualifications.
The situation is different in most countries of Europe,
where only registered medical practitioners may practise
any form of medicine, and the legal framework for CAM
is much more restrictive (Sheldon 2004).

The revised UK Medical Act passed in 1858, while
continuing to link the initial license to practise with
graduation from a university, created the framework
whereby conventional medicine could essentially govern
itself under legal authority of the State. A statutory
regulatory body, the General Medical Council, came into
being, and was given authority to license and register
practitioners, to set standards for practice, to control medical
education and training through inspection and accreditation
of medical schools, and to conduct disciplinary proceedings
against doctors if necessary. National health services would
only employ doctors who were registered with the GMC,
and removal from the GMC register equated to loss of the
right to practise as a doctor in the UK. Thus, the GMC was
granted very considerable powers over individual doctors
and over the medical profession collectively, and became
generally accountable to the public for standards of medical
practice in the UK.

Subsequently, systems for the state-approved licensing
and registration of other conventional healthcare practitioners
were introduced, initially to include nurses, midwives,
dentists and opticians. For example, the Royal College
of Nursing was established in 1916 for this purpose.
The Professions Supplementary to Medicine Act 1960
created similar arrangements for physiotherapists,
occupational therapists, radiographers, dietitians,
chiropodists and medical laboratory scientific officers.
As part of this 1960 Act, the Council for Professions
Supplementary to Medicine was established, with functions
analogous to those of the General Medical Council, and with
strong medical representation on the Council. Again, only
those healthcare professionals who were licensed and
registered with the Council were eligible for employment
in the National Health Service.

Such systems for professional licensing and registration,
linked to regulation of standards of practice, are of value
in that they help to protect patients from incompetent and
potentially dangerous practitioners – although events such
as the Shipman Inquiry indicate that they are not always
wholly effective in this regard. They also help to identify
professional status and create communities of practice with
shared values and common goals, who can support each
other when required. At the same time, they establish
boundaries between professions, which may allow
professional groupings to develop exclusive rights and
protect their own interests. Conversely, the lack of state-
approved statutory licensing, registration and regulation
of practice for most forms of CAM may influence the way
in which CAM is regarded by patients, by the National
Health Service, and by conventional medical practitioners
(Fig. 7). It also creates a context where any conventional
healthcare provider may choose to combine conventional
and alternative practice, as is commonly seen in Europe,
China and elsewhere. Thus, increasingly there is a trend

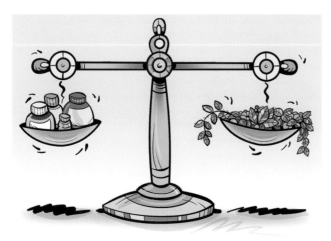

Fig. 7 **Conventional and complementary medicine are constantly being 'weighed in the balance' by patients, by the state, and by practitioners of both types.** A relative lack of professional regulation inevitably influences the way in which CAM is viewed.

towards systems for registration and regulation of CAM practitioners.

The most advanced of the CAM therapies in this respect are osteopathy and chiropractic. Both of these are subject to similar Acts of Parliament, passed in 1993 and 1994, which established professional regulatory councils, and limited the right to use the title of osteopath or chiropractor to practitioners who are registered with them. There is a striking similarity between the aims, constitution and modus operandi of the General Osteopathic Council and

---

Table 6 **Professional regulation in osteopathy (http://www.osteopathy.org.uk/)**

The aims of the General Osteopathic Council are:
- to protect patients
- to develop the osteopathic profession
- to promote an understanding of osteopathic care.

The Council:
- registers qualified professionals
- sets standards for osteopathic practice and conduct
- assures the quality of osteopathic education
- ensures continuing professional development
- helps patients with complaints about an osteopath.

Case study

A review of the issues relating to professional regulation and educational standards for CAM practitioners by Mills (2001) stated:
- 'Practitioners of complementary and alternative medicine in the United Kingdom are free to practice as they wish.'
- 'Most therapies have set up professional bodies, but the educational standards required by these bodies vary widely.'
- 'House of Lords recently reviewed complementary and alternative medicine and recommended clearer regulation.'
- 'Because of the wide variation in therapies, each discipline should initially set up its own regulatory body, although it may be possible to combine these later.'
- 'Many patients consult complementary practitioners without telling their doctor, with possible detrimental effects on health care; greater cooperation and respect between orthodox and complementary practitioners would improve communication with patients.'

---

those of the General Medical Council (Table 6). There is fairly general agreement that a similar regulatory framework for other forms of complementary medicine is desirable (Mills 2001a). As described later in this text in the chapters related to individual therapies, many groups of CAM practitioners have organised themselves into professional associations. In general, however, these lack official legal status, are not formally approved by the state, and cannot confer rights to employment by the National Health Service. In some cases a number of different bodies exist in relation to a particular therapy. It should be noted that many CAM therapists practise more than one, and often several, forms of treatment. Opponents of statutory regulation refer to the holistic nature of complementary medical practice, which focuses on the needs of the patient in the widest sense, and is often not confined to the diagnosis and treatment of a specific disease or condition. Thus it is argued that regulatory systems and processes which replicate the rigid requirements of conventional medicine are unnecessary, and would in any case be extremely difficult to implement and sustain (Stone & Matthews 1996).

As one potential solution, it has been proposed that CAM practitioners could be included in the provisions of the Professions Supplementary to Medicine Act 1960 (see above). Registration under the Act would bring entitlement to employment within the National Health Service. However, at the present time it is unclear how many complementary practitioners, given the option, would choose to work within the highly regulated, supervised and primarily biomedical framework of the NHS. Registration under the Act is not relevant to issues of professional practice in the private sector. The view has been expressed that any advantages to CAM practitioners of registration under the 1960 Act and the Council for Professions Supplementary to Medicine would be outweighed by a loss of professional autonomy and independence (Stone & Matthews 1996). These debates continue actively; it remains uncertain to what extent CAM will move from what is primarily a system of voluntary self-regulation towards a formal regulatory framework authorised and recognised by the state. It seems unlikely that a single system will be found which can deal effectively with the number and diversity of complementary therapies which currently exist.

Relationships between conventional and CAM practice

As a result of increasing patient demand and the moves towards regulation in some parts of the CAM community, CAM services are increasingly available either within the National Health Service or in very close relationship to it (Dobson 2003). There are various ways in which this relationship may operate (Table 7).

Table 7 **Relationships between CAM and orthodox medical practice**

- Individual practitioners who practise both CAM and orthodox medicine. Because of the regulation issue, this is almost always in the form of a conventional practitioner who also delivers CAM services, rather than the converse.
- Conventional and CAM services being delivered side-by-side in hospital units or general practice, in an integrated service, but by separate practitioners.
- The referral/delegation of patients by conventional practitioners to CAM therapists. This may or may not be funded by the NHS.

Such relationships raise important issues concerning accountability, autonomy and clinical decision-making. For example, the situation when a conventional medical practitioner requests the involvement of a CAM therapist in the care of a patient is less than clear. Is this 'referral' or 'delegation'? *Referral* implies that while the referring practitioner retains some clinical responsibility for the patient, the practitioner receiving the referral will assume full professional and legal liability for the care that they give. *Delegation* indicates that the delegating professional remains accountable for all of the treatment provided to 'their' patient. In the case of CAM treatments, it is questionable whether doctors can reasonably be held accountable for the outcome of therapies which they may not fully understand, where the evidence for efficacy in conventional biomedical terms may be weak or absent, or where the professional standing and licensure status of the provider may not be explicit. Thus the process is most accurately described as referral, although the Department of Health in 1991 issued guidance to the contrary. This issue remains unclear legally and professionally, and may represent a barrier to meaningful integration of healthcare provision.

When conventional doctors practise a CAM therapy, they:

- should undertake recognised training in that field, approved by the appropriate regulatory body
- should only practise the therapy after registration
- are accountable to the General Medical Council for any treatment they administer
- have a responsibility to maintain their continuing professional development in all the areas of their clinical practice
- should participate in audit and related clinical governance activities.

Source: British Medical Association (1999).

Conventional perspectives on CAM

Different approaches to understanding health and illness

Michael T. Ross

This section explores some of the issues surrounding CAM from a Western medical perspective in the first few years of the 21st century. Such perspectives are neither static nor standardised, as therapies and approaches to healthcare go in and out of fashion over time and vary widely between countries and cultures. If a treatment is not part of mainstream healthcare in any given culture it is defined as CAM; if it subsequently becomes mainstream it will cease to be CAM and will become 'conventional'. Historians are starting to explore this phenomenon and highlight the importance of culture, public opinion, financial interests and political manoeuvring in delineating the boundaries of conventional medicine (Saks 1996, Porter 1988). CAM therapies are frequently discussed in the media, where there is a tendency for them to be portrayed with sweeping generalisations and emotive headlines (Fig. 8). Such

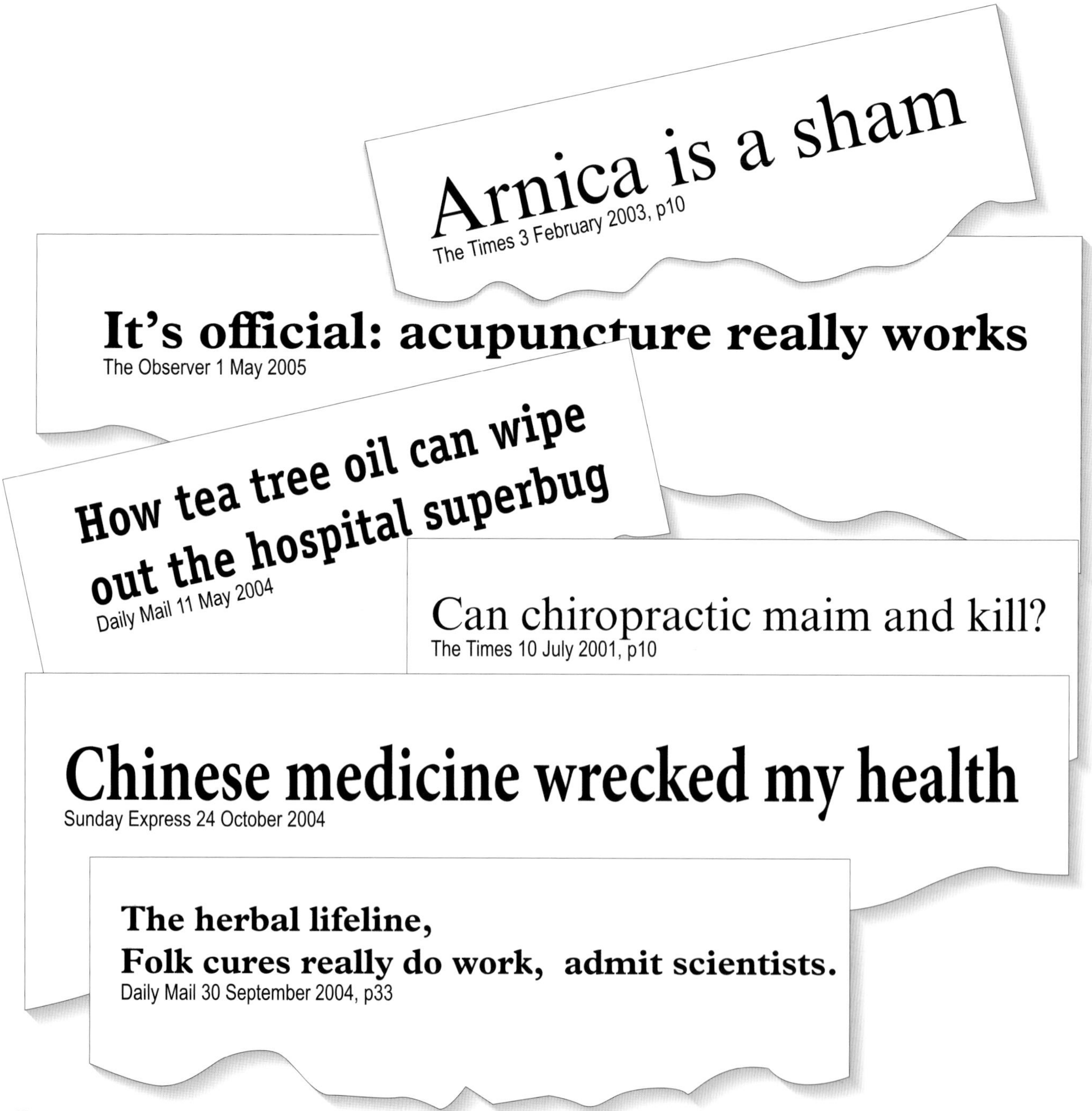

Arnica is a sham
The Times 3 February 2003, p10

It's official: acupuncture really works
The Observer 1 May 2005

How tea tree oil can wipe out the hospital superbug
Daily Mail 11 May 2004

Can chiropractic maim and kill?
The Times 10 July 2001, p10

Chinese medicine wrecked my health
Sunday Express 24 October 2004

The herbal lifeline,
Folk cures really do work, admit scientists.
Daily Mail 30 September 2004, p33

Fig. 8 **Media headlines on CAM.**

reporting can significantly influence the views of health professionals as well as those of the general public. Issues raised in the popular press are now often discussed with the evidence in medical journals and websites such as the 'hitting the headlines' section of the NHS E-library (www/nelh.nhs.uk/hth/archive.asp). Such resources can be particularly useful when patients wish to discuss something they have read or heard about on radio or television with their doctor.

This book aims to convey the message that CAM approaches should neither be unquestioningly accepted nor automatically disregarded. To consider classes of CAM as a collective entity to accept or reject would be akin to making this type of polarised judgement on the practice of surgery or all conventional medicines. CAM is a very complex and diverse field and each therapy is likely to have merits and demerits – not least in terms of efficacy and safety.

Conventional Western perspective on efficacy, safety and evidence

Following the work of Archie Cochrane in the 1970s and the Evidence Based Medicine (EBM) working group in the 1990s, most Western countries have adopted the concept that all healthcare decisions should be guided by the best available scientific evidence. Previously clinicians would have relied more exclusively upon experience, logic and advice from others, and policy-makers would have relied upon the balance of specialist opinions and available resources (Gray 1997). Increasingly evidence is being sought to support or reject all aspects of conventional medical activity including prevention, screening, diagnosis, treatment and policy-making (Sackett et al 2000).

This 'evidence-based' approach is now being applied, rightly or wrongly, to homeopathy, osteopathy, acupuncture and even intercessory prayer. In this way a degree of efficacy has been demonstrated for a small number of specific CAM approaches such as acupressure for nausea and vomiting in pregnancy, fish oil supplements for rheumatoid arthritis and hypercholesterolaemia, and St John's wort for depression (SCHIN 2002). The number of high-quality CAM studies conducted using a conventional EBM approach is small but increasing and many conventional health professionals now view treatments validated in this way as useful tools in the therapeutic armoury. For some CAM therapies such as acupuncture or spinal manipulation for chronic asthma evidence suggests they are ineffective and may even be harmful, (SCHIN 2002, SIGN-BTS 2004). Even without such evidence, most conventional doctors would also be very concerned about their patient taking traditional Chinese medicines containing arsenic and mercury or declining surgery for their cancer in preference for osteopathy. For the majority of CAM therapies, however, there is no clear evidence of efficacy and opinions vary widely, ranging from mistrust and avoidance to daily use depending upon past experience and familiarity.

Conventional and CAM perspectives on health and illness

The EBM approach is based on conventional Western diagnoses, which in turn are based on a Western scientific understanding of health and illness. There are, however, fundamental differences of opinion on the causes of ill health and diagnostic processes between conventional medicine and various types of CAM. How then can doctors apply Western concepts of efficacy and evidence to CAM therapies without agreement on the condition being treated? When looking at the evidence for CAM it is therefore helpful to avoid considering them purely as therapeutics, but rather whole approaches to health, illness and healing. Healthcare professionals need to be familiar with the variety of approaches used within a multicultural society.

Different approaches to health and illness

1. Biomedical approaches
Western diagnoses and concepts of health and illness stem from an understanding of biomedical sciences such as anatomy and physiology, the roots of which can be traced back via the Belgian anatomist and physician Andreas Vesalius (1514–1564 AD; Fig. 9) to the ancient Greek Hippocrates (460–377 BC). A typical biomedical Western consultation consists of gathering information, diagnosing and addressing the problem(s) (Fig. 10).

2. Holistic approaches
Ancient Chinese philosophers and healers also studied people in great depth but in a different way and arrived at a completely different understanding of how parts of the body are connected together and interact, and of the

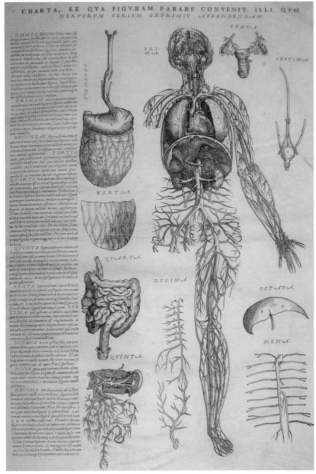

Fig. 9 **Vesalius (1514–1564).** (Reproduced with kind permission of Glasgow University Library Special Collections.)

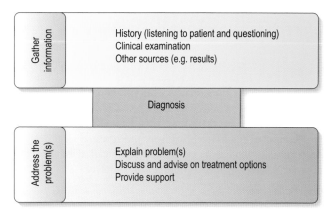

Fig. 10 **Simplified Western biomedical approach to illness.**

nature of the mind/body/spirit interface. For example, an understanding of the channels and flow of qi (chi) around the body (Fig. 11) underpins many Eastern CAM therapies including acupuncture, reflexology and t'ai chi. No anatomical structures have been identified by dissection or microscopy to account for these channels, although localised concentrations of nerves, vessels and metabolic activity at acupuncture points have been described (Wei et al 1999). Other cultures have also studied the mind/body/spirit interface and 'holistic' approaches to health and illness, developing understandings of the body which are different again, such as the seven wheels or 'chakras' of reiki (Fig. 12), the principles of Indian Ayurveda and many others.

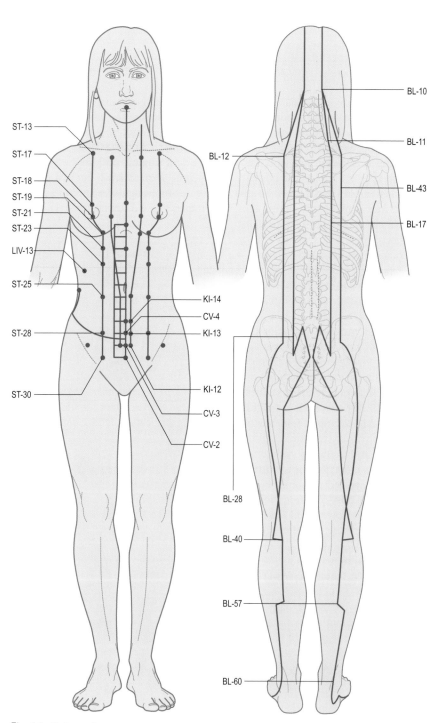

Fig. 11 **Qi channels.**

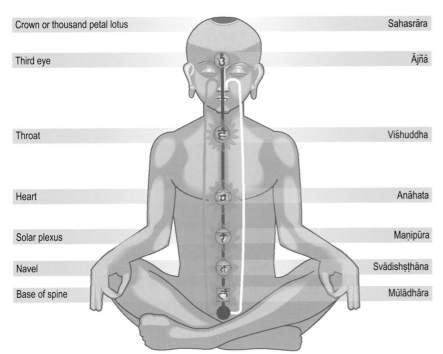

Crown or thousand petal lotus	Sahasrāra	Fig. 12 **Chakras.**
Third eye	Ājñā	
Throat	Viśhuddha	
Heart	Anāhata	
Solar plexus	Maṇipūra	
Navel	Svādishṭhāna	
Base of spine	Mūlādhāra	

3. Deontological approaches

The third approach explains health and illness in terms of external spiritual or deontological forces acting on the body. It is likely that such beliefs about health and illness have been more prevalent throughout history in both primitive and modern societies than either biomedical or holistic models. Health is seen as a gift from God. Illness can be seen as the result of competing influences of good and evil (Fig. 13) and/or as the result of sin – either personal wrongdoings, or more generally. Healing may be brought about by prayer, faith, sacrifice or gaining favour with God(s). Although some of these are human actions, practitioners do not believe the actions directly cause healing, but rather appeal to God(s) to intervene on their behalf.

4. Implications in practice

An individual disabled with painful swollen joints going to practitioners of each of these three approaches in turn could be diagnosed as having rheumatoid arthritis, a blockage of qi in the joints caused by the external factors of cold and damp (Mills 1988) and being bound by evil forces (Luke 13:10–17 NIV). These diagnoses are not as mutually incompatible as they may at first seem and it is quite possible that each is simply a partial view of the patient's true condition. Management of the patient by practitioners of each approach would clearly be quite different, however, and may include the disease-modifying drug azathioprine, acupuncture and prayer respectively. Because the diagnoses and outcomes are so diverse, it is difficult to compare the efficacy or even safety of these treatments. If a controlled trial was attempted the population would have to consist of individuals with exactly the same bio-psycho-socio-spiritual condition, rather than simply a population of individuals with rheumatoid arthritis.

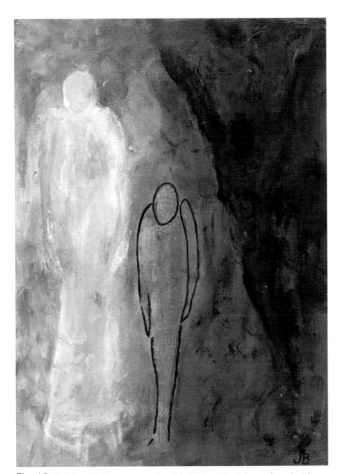

Fig. 13 **Spiritual influences on health.** ('Who Wins?' Reproduced with kind permission of Justin Baldwins, artist.)

Summary

- Anything that is not 'conventional' medicine is defined as CAM and the boundaries between these are in constant flux.
- There are fundamental differences in understanding of health and illness between conventional medicine and many types of CAM.
- Different perspectives and approaches to health and illness can be roughly categorised as biomedical, holistic, deontological or combinations of these.

■ Therapies cannot be directly compared without agreement on the problem being treated and the outcome measures sought.

STOP THINK
■ What therapies do you know that used to be considered CAM but are now considered conventional medicine?
■ Have you ever met two or more people in whom a disease was expressed in exactly the same way and who also had the same bio-psycho-socio-spiritual co-morbidity?

Different approaches to treating and preventing illness

Michael T. Ross

It is helpful to explore different ways of looking at therapeutic effectiveness in clinical practice and some approaches to illness prevention and health promotion, both in conventional medicine and in CAM. Factors contributing to overall effectiveness in treating illness can be divided into three domains of efficacy, consultation factors and suitability – each of which are amenable to different types of investigation and research (Fig. 14). Some factors contributing to therapeutic effectiveness also apply to preventive healthcare measures and health promotion. Each of these will be considered separately with examples from conventional medicine and CAM.

Factors contributing to effectiveness in treating illness

1. Efficacy

Efficacy is 'the ability of an intervention to produce the desired beneficial effect in expert hands and under ideal circumstances' (Newman Dorland 2000). The term is often used interchangeably with the more general 'effectiveness' but they have subtly different meanings when used in a medical context (Fig. 15). Paracetamol has been shown to be a more efficacious analgesic than placebo in blinded randomised controlled trials (Arendt-Nielson et al 1991),

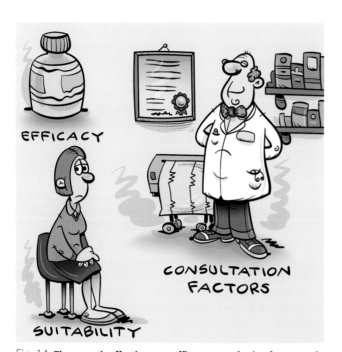

Fig. 14 **Therapeutic effectiveness: efficacy, consultation factors and suitability.**

efficacy: 1. *The ability of an intervention to produce the desired effect in expert hands and under ideal circumstances.*
2. *In pharmacology, the ability of a drug to produce the desired therapeutic effect.*

effectiveness: 1. *The ability to produce a specific result or to exert a specific measurable influence.*
2. *The ability of an intervention to produce the desired beneficial effect in actual use.*

i.e. 'efficacy' is the inherent pharmacological or other properties which influence outcomes when consultation factors (ideal circumstances) and suitability to the individual patient (expert hands) are controlled-for, as in clinical trials.
Effectiveness relates to more general outcomes when using a particular treatment in clinical practice which result from the combined effects and interactions of all of these factors.

Newman Dorlan 2000

Fig. 15 **Definitions of efficacy and effectiveness from *Dorland's Illustrated Medical Dictionary.*** (Newman Dorland 2000).

and is often helpful even in sceptical patients irrespective of whether they get it from a doctor or local garage. There is currently considerable interest in demonstrating such efficacy for specific CAM therapies. St John's Wort, for example, has been shown to be more efficacious than placebo in treating depression (Linde et al 1996) and at least as efficacious and better tolerated than paroxetine (Szegedi et al 2005) and imipramine (Woelk 2000). In many such studies a conventional biomedical diagnosis is made without input from a trained herbalist and patients are randomly allocated to each treatment group to reduce consultation factors and possible selection bias.

2. Consultation factors

Any interaction with a patient can be considered to be a 'consultation'. The therapeutic potential of the consultation itself has been studied extensively in conventional medicine, and the importance of environmental, communication and other factors on patient outcomes has been demonstrated (Neighbour 2004, Tate 2003). There is also some evidence suggesting that the duration and timing of a consultation, the room environment, the therapist's clothing and even their accent may also have a considerable effect on clinical outcomes. Many people consider these factors influence outcomes via the 'placebo effect', which is the name given to the phenomenon whereby individuals who expect clinical improvement from an intervention achieve better clinical outcomes (Beecher 1955, Kirsch & Sapirstein 1998). It relates to patient attitudes and expectations of therapies rather than efficacy. 'Placebo' treatments are inactive simulations of real treatments, common examples being sugar tablets which look identical to medicinal products and sham acupuncture outside known points or with non-piercing needles (Fink et al 2001, Lewith et al 2002). Study patients in placebo-controlled trials consent to receiving placebo or active treatments, and the effects of active treatment are only thought to be significant if they are better than placebo. Patients in clinical trials typically do not know whether they are receiving active treatment or placebo (called a 'blind' trial). Clinicians delivering treatment or collecting results will often not know either (a 'double-blind' trial), although it is not always possible to blind the therapist, as in sham acupuncture.

Whilst patients can give consent for active or placebo treatments in clinical trials, by definition they cannot give informed consent for placebo use in clinical practice. Many Western clinicians reject their use in practice on ethical grounds, although they are still used in some countries (Nitzan & Lichtenberg 2004). The placebo effect, however, is likely to be a feature of all healthcare interactions with patients, exerting more or less influence on outcomes depending upon how closely the consultation and therapist meet with patient expectations and how much confidence they have that the therapy will improve their condition. Such consultation factors will also have a considerable influence on patient anxiety, recall of information and concordance with recommended medication and lifestyle changes.

3. Suitability

Even if a therapy has proven efficacy for the patient's condition and consultation factors are optimal, treatments that are effective for one patient may not be suitable for another even though in some respects the patients have a similar illness. The conventional antibiotic trimethoprim, for example, has demonstrable efficacy in treating many but not all urine infections (SCHIN 2002). The conventional scientific explanation is that not all bacteria which can cause a urine infection are sensitive to this antibiotic, and so further information is required (sending urine to a laboratory for culture and testing of antibiotic sensitivity) to help tailor antibiotic therapy to the individual patient.

In addition to this biological suitability, there is also growing literature on the importance of other aspects, such as the patient's narrative in Western conventional 'narrative-based medicine' (Greenhalgh 1999). By exploring patients' own 'narratives' about their illness and identifying their ideas, concerns and expectations, subsequent explanation, advice and treatment can be tailored more appropriately, resulting in better clinical outcomes. For example, antidepressants and psychological therapy have been shown to be effective in treating depression, but teaching relaxation techniques and offering practical help with social and financial issues may actually lead to better outcomes in some individuals. CAM practitioners also gather additional information to help tailor their choice of therapies to individual patients. Homeopaths identify highly individual patterns of symptoms and signs and select active ingredients which, if given in high dose, would most closely produce a similar illness. Herbalists, osteopaths and acupuncturists select therapies based on a holistic assessment of the patient's illness. Aromatherapists may offer a range of suitable essential oils which may be suitable, allowing patients to select those they prefer. As many of these treatments are very patient-specific, the effectiveness of such approaches is more likely to be appreciated in qualitative studies rather than quantitative controlled trials.

Effectiveness in preventing illness

> Prevention is better than cure. (Desiderius Erasmus 1466–1536)

A significant proportion of the UK budget is spent on preventing illness. Some of this "preventative medicine" is delivered by doctors to individual patients by vaccination (against serious infections such as measles, meningitis C and tuberculosis), screening for early disease (e.g. antenatal, child development, cervical and breast screening), health promotion (such as exercise and smoking cessation) and preventing the deterioration of established diseases (such as asthma, coronary heart disease and diabetes). It is likely that the majority of disease, however, is prevented by general health education; legislation to ensure clean drinking water; safer foods, electrical appliances and road travel; pest control and customs regulations; the notification and contact tracing of infectious diseases; employment law; environmental policies; and controls on drugs, tobacco and alcohol. Even apparently small changes in legislation can have large effects on population health, such as reducing the number of fatal paracetamol overdoses by restricting pack sizes available without prescription (Hawton et al 2004). Such measures to prevent illness, although not directly visible to patients attending their doctor, are nevertheless a result of better understanding of health and disease from the scientific Western perspective and are heavily influenced by public health doctors. It is the large body of research connecting tobacco smoking with lung cancer and other illnesses in both active and passive smokers that has led to global anti-smoking strategies and the prohibition of smoking in enclosed public workplaces such as bars and restaurants in Ireland, the UK and elsewhere (Shibuya et al 2003, Howell 2004). The effectiveness of such preventive strategies can be studied by looking prospectively at outcome measures in whole populations over both the short term (studies of morbidity such as respiratory tract infections and absence from work) and the long term (morbidity and mortality from vascular disease and cancer).

The prevention of illness is also a dominant feature of most CAM. As with conventional Western doctors, many CAM practitioners will advise individuals on healthy living with plenty of exercise, a balanced healthy diet with adequate vitamins and minerals, a sensible alcohol intake and regular sleep and relaxation. There is growing evidence for the effectiveness of such preventive lifestyle changes (SCHIN 2002). However, CAM therapists may also advise unconventional health promotion measures such as rearranging living spaces for maximal balance of qi with feng shui; to walk, sit and lift items in a particular way with Alexander technique; or to meditate or perform repetitive exercise activities such as yoga or t'ai chi. They may advise regular therapies such as herbal teas, mega-vitamin and herbal supplements, radically altering the diet, inhaling incense or aromatherapy vapours and the consumption of a variety of unconventional medicines and products. A few recommend that subjects receive intermittent preventive therapy administered by the practitioner in person over long periods. As with all preventive healthcare measures, the outcomes are often multifactorial and difficult to study, although studies of primary and secondary prevention using CAM are beginning to appear in the literature. *Ginkgo biloba* has been shown to arrest cognitive decline in patients diagnosed with dementia (Le Bars et al 1997), Catholic rosary prayers and yogic mantras have been shown to

■ What consultation factors might maximise the 'placebo effect', and how might these differ between conventional and CAM consultations?
■ Think about some health promotion or preventive strategies that are based on Western biomedical approaches to health and illness. How might these differ in societies with holistic or deontological approaches?

optimise autonomic cardiovascular rhythms (Bernardi et al 2001) and regular consumption of certain mega-dose vitamins has been shown to be harmful (Expert Group on Vitamins and Minerals 2003). As well as using traditional Chinese medicine alongside modern 'conventional' medicine in the Chinese healthcare system, there are also separate departments of traditional medicine in the Ministry and local Bureaux of Public Health (Hesketh & Zhu 1997), influencing health promotion and illness prevention on a population scale.

Summary

■ CAM therapies are amenable to scientific studies of efficacy.
■ Factors contributing to the effectiveness of a therapy in clinical practice can be considered under therapeutic efficacy, consultation factors and individual suitability.
■ Most health promotion and illness preventive measures in the UK are based on Western biomedical perspectives on health and illness, but this may not be the case in other societies and cultures.

Safety of complementary and alternative medicines

Michael T. Ross

"It is to be much regretted, that medicines thus offered to the public are not by appointment of the legislature examined by persons properly qualified to ascertain their inefficacy or utility. That on one hand, an useful discovery might not be disregarded as the imposition of a quack; and on the other, that the weak and credulous might not be defrauded of their money for something that is useless, if not hurtful to their health." (Source: **Gentleman's magazine** *1734 4:818; quoted in Porter 1988)*

Most criticisms of CAM from conventional medical practitioners relate to concerns about safety. Such concerns are not new or unique to CAM, and may be frequently exaggerated. Perhaps because many CAM therapies have previously been thought of as harmless, and partly because of a general lack of understanding, any reports of side effects or interactions of individual CAM therapies may bias individuals' views of entire CAM fields. A common example of such a response by some Westerners is a total mistrust of all traditional Chinese medicine because some have been found to contain undeclared, potentially harmful ingredients.

Safety aspects of conventional medicine

Conventional medicines, whether prescribed or not, are now packaged with patient information leaflets containing lists of known side effects and interactions with other medicines (BMA & RPSGB 2005). Minor side effects are not uncommon with conventional medicines and severe reactions do sometimes occur. There are also well-known complications and undesirable effects associated with surgical treatments, physiotherapy manipulations and even some lifestyle changes. Conventional medicine cannot in any way be considered totally safe. Doctors and other therapists learn about the potential side effects and complications of their therapies, however, are obliged to share this information with patients so they can make 'informed decisions' about their own health (GMC 1998).

Regulation and safety aspects of CAM therapies

CAM therapists are not currently obliged to share information about the potential harmful effects of their treatments in the same way as conventional practitioners, even if they are aware of common adverse outcomes, largely due to heterogeneity and lack of regulation within professional bodies.

Most CAM therapies have not been regarded by law as 'medicines' and have not required the same evidence of effectiveness as conventional therapeutic agents. Most CAM products were not regulated as medicines by the Medicines Act 1968. They have been regarded as foods, and as such, were subject to the much less stringent Food Safety Act 1990, Food Labelling Regulations 1996, Trade Descriptions Act 1968 and more recently the EU Directive 2002/46/EC on food supplements (Council Directive 2002).

Herbal remedies were specifically exempt from the Medicines Act 1968 (section 12) as long as they were made by drying, crushing or comminuting a plant or plants on the premises, to be sold after a consultation, without written indications, and not carrying a trade name other than the plant(s) and process used. This situation is changing with new European legislation on herbal medicines and other CAM, coordinated by the European Agency for the Evaluation of Medicinal Products (EMEA). It is likely that CAM therapies will soon be subject to similar standards as conventional medicines.

Safety issues for specific CAM therapies

The UK government Medicines and Healthcare Products Regulatory Agency (MHRA) publishes reports on adverse effects, interactions and other safety issues of medicines, and has legal powers to act on such information to prevent further harm. Similar bodies exist in other countries, such as the FDA Med-Watch monitoring system in the United States. Much of their evidence is collected from individual reports, and in the United Kingdom these are usually submitted by professionals via the 'yellow card' notification system.

Doctors, pharmacists and most other conventional health professionals are aware of the yellow card system and would use it for this purpose. Members of the public can now also submit their own reports directly, which the MHRA will act upon. CAM practitioners can also use this reporting system and the collected reports, although at present there are infrequent contributions relating to CAM. Data collected in this way are collated systematically and listed alphabetically by drug on the yellow card website (www.yellowcard.gov.uk). Those listed currently include evening primrose oil, *Hypericum perforatum*, rock rose flower extract (in Rescue Remedy), and menthol. There are currently 190 reports of adverse effects for menthol, with 4 suspected fatal outcomes. The MHRA website also has several pages dedicated to herbal medicine called 'Herbal Safety News', which is the source of many of the serious documented harmful effects of CAM detailed in Table 8. Many of the more minor side effects (such as vasovagal faints with acupuncture and allergic reactions with herbal medicine) and those which relate to physical therapies (such as soft tissue damage in osteopathy or skin irritation from aromatherapy) will not be listed on the MHRA site, but the better specialist CAM textbooks will contain such information (Barnes et al 1996).

Table 8 **Some mechanisms by which CAM can be harmful**

1. Source of infection
Examples:
- Chinese medicine Nu Bao containing human placenta
- Acupuncture using non-sterile needles (Ernst & White 1997)

2. Directly harmful ingredients or practices
Examples:
- Heavy metals mercury, lead and arsenic found in the Ayurvedic medicine Muhayogaraj Guggulu
- Plant toxins aconite (Dickens et al 1994), *Aristolochia* and kava-kava
- Irritation and photosensitivity from essential oils and *Psoralea* fruit extracts
- Specific risks if used during pregnancy or lactation, e.g. ginseng which has been shown to be teratogenic in rats
- Risk of physical trauma such as pneumothorax and cardiac tamponade from acupuncture (Vincent 2001)
- Risk of nerve damage from neck manipulation (Stevinson et al 2001).

3. Poor professional standards and inadequate regulation
- Variability in the training, qualifications and governance of CAM. Can assume the role and title of CAM practitioner after little or no training, with the exceptions of osteopathy and chiropractic (www.dh.gov.uk)
- Serious conventional illnesses such as asthma or cancer may be inadequately investigated or treated (SCHIN 2002)
- Poor labelling with variable contents, concentrations and quantities, or containing the wrong ingredient, e.g. *Podophyllum* substituted for gentian, digitalis for plantain and *Teucrium* for *Scutellaria*
- Inadequate restriction on advertising and claims of safety and effectiveness
- May contain Western prescription-only medicines (POM) such as corticosteroids, sildenafil in the Chinese medicines Hua Fo and Wei Ge Wang; glibenclamide (anti-diabetic) in Xiaoke-Wan; paracetamol, diclofenac and antihistamine in Shu Xiao Shang Feng (Ministry of Health, New Zealand 2003).

4. Lack of public understanding about CAM
- May be considered 'safe' and 'harmless' by the public, so increased risk of poor concordance or accidental overdose
- Many CAM therapies interact with Western medication (e.g. St John's wort)
- Patients may not tell their doctor or CAM therapist about other treatments
- Dietary changes may cause significant harm through interactions with medication, such as cranberry with warfarin or grapefruit with statins
- Certain CAM medicines may cause problems during surgery due to interactions or effects on clotting and blood pressure (e.g. garlic, ginseng and ginkgo)
- Accidental or misinformed ingestion of toxic aromatherapy essential oils.

Source: MHRA website (accessed June, 2006) unless otherwise stated.

■ How can you tell if a CAM practitioner has undergone any professional training and is practising the standard one would expect of a healthcare professional?

■ What was the last drug side effect or interaction you saw? Was it reported to the MHRA?

Summary

■ As with conventional therapies, CAM is not totally harmless.
■ All suspected adverse effects or interactions of conventional medicines or CAM should be reported to the MHRA,

allowing them to investigate and act to prevent further harm and also enhancing the usefulness of their collected resource.

Sources of further information

■ Department of Health: www.dh.gov.uk
■ European Agency for the Evaluation of Medicinal Products: www.emea.eu.int
■ General Chiropractic Council: www.gcc-uk.org
■ General Osteopathic Council: www.osteopathy.org.uk
■ MHRA – Medicines and Healthcare Products Regulatory Agency: www.mhra.gov.uk
■ RPSGB – Royal Pharmaceutical Society of Great Britain: www.rpsgb.org

Finding evidence for CAM

Marshal F. Dozier

Patients are becoming more informed, more questioning and more direct in relation to their own healthcare. Self-help groups and sources of high-quality patient information abound, and some individuals are becoming recognised as 'expert patients' – people who have a particular long-term condition and can use their experience and knowledge to help others (exemplified by the UK National Health Service Expert Patients Programme – www.expertpatients.nhs.uk), and this is definitely to be encouraged. A result, though, is that even if conventional medical practitioners try to avoid CAM, it is likely that sooner or later patients will ask their opinions about it anyway. This section covers how to approach finding evidence for the effectiveness of CAM. As we describe each step in the process, we refer to the example scenario presented in the Case study 'Finding evidence step by step', and continues in the next section – 'Assessing evidence for quality and relevance'.

Case study

Finding evidence step by step

Scenario
A 35-year-old woman presents to her doctor with ongoing depression. She has stopped her antidepressant (fluoxetine) because of side effects and asks about St John's wort. The doctor is aware of conflicting information on the efficacy of St John's wort and potential interactions with conventional antidepressants.

Sample research question
How does St John's wort compare with serotonin uptake inhibitors in terms of effectiveness and safety in the treatment of moderate depression?

Ask an answerable question

Before setting out to find evidence for the safety, benefits or harm of CAM therapies (or any therapy), it is helpful to formulate a focused clinical query that captures the salient elements of the patient's situation. Sackett's 'PICO' model (Sackett et al 2000) can make this easier:

■ **P**atient or population: what are the defining features of the patient's illness and background?
■ **I**ntervention: what is the therapeutic intervention or exposure being assessed?
■ **C**omparison: are you comparing the intervention with another intervention or placebo?
■ **O**utcome(s): what measurable outcomes are you looking for?

The PICO format is particularly useful for questions about therapeutic effectiveness, but it may be necessary to find other types of information – such as aetiology, diagnosis, epidemiology or prognosis of a condition – to place the information in context.

The case study illustrates this step with a research question that is used to capture the essential elements presented in the scenario: moderate depression (patient); St John's Wort (intervention); serotonin uptake inhibitors (comparison); effectiveness and safety (outcomes).

In shaping the question on therapeutic effectiveness, it can help to establish whether the issue is about disease prevention or cure, or improvement in quality of life in patients in rehabilitation or with chronic or terminal conditions.

By identifying the type(s) of research methodology that will yield the data required to answer the question at the outset (e.g. randomised controlled trial, cohort study, focus group), it is easier to filter out irrelevant reports and more difficult to be distracted by studies that do not address the issues in the question. The methods of measuring the outcomes of an intervention can usually help to define the most appropriate research methodology.

It is essential to take an unbiased approach to finding evidence: the expectation of finding positive reports on the safety and effectiveness of an intervention makes a searcher more likely to see and select only positive reports from the body of search results. The searcher must be sure to look for reports of positive, negative or neutral results.

Searching for evidence

At the time of writing, there are well over 700 000 web pages about St John's wort and depression, of variable quality. However, the sources of further information listed give a selection of high-quality internet-based resources that should give good coverage for most CAM. Literature databases usually only contain bibliographic details of journal articles, books or reports, and although some have links to the full text, it will generally be necessary to use a library to find the complete publication. The key CAM resources on the net provide references and often have links to bibliographic databases, but generally have a lot of useful information on the websites themselves.

The type of information required to answer the research question will help to determine the resources that should be searched. The scenario and research question presented in our example are best answered by studies that measure St John's wort against fluoxetine or other serotonin uptake inhibitors (like controlled trials), or analyses that synthesise multiple comparable studies (systematic reviews, perhaps with meta-analyses). It is more efficient and reliable to take advantage of good quality systematic reviews than to search for and compare controlled trials. Clinical guidelines based on systematic reviews of evidence are also a good place to look.

Figure 16 shows a search of each subject with synonyms in the Medline database. The number of publications retrieved with each search is shown in the right-hand column. It is easy to see how the number of results is reduced when all the subjects are combined together. In the last line of the search history, the results are further limited by a ready-made clinical query filter for therapeutic effectiveness that isolates results about clinical trials. Bear in mind that this search filter is oriented toward the randomised controlled trial, which may not always be appropriate.

Literature searching is usually an iterative process (Fig. 17). It is normal to adjust an initial research question on the basis of information found after one or two searches. Sometimes it is necessary to broaden a search because too little information is retrieved. To broaden a search, try including synonyms or more general – but still relevant – concepts (Fig. 18). For example, if the sample search were on all antidepressant agents instead of fluoxetine and other serotonin uptake inhibitors, the number of results in the sample search would more than triple. Conversely, sometimes it is necessary to narrow the scope of the question because an unmanageable amount of information is retrieved (Fig. 19). To narrow a search, think about choosing more precise search terms or including additional required concepts.

Summary

- There is a variety of sources of information for CAM. The decision on which one(s) to use should be based on the type of evidence required (Fig. 20).
- Finding evidence is more efficient when the searcher starts by creating a focused research question (Fig. 21).
- The focused research question should take an unbiased approach to positive or negative reports of effectiveness.
- The key concepts in the research question can be used as initial search terms. The search terms may be refined as the search progresses.

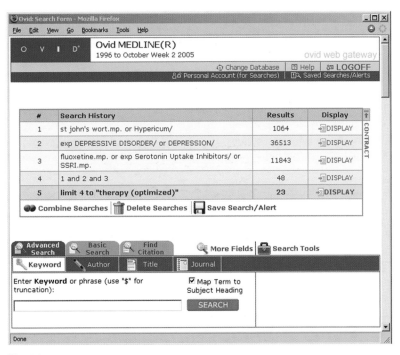

Fig. 16 **Medline search output.** (Courtesy of Medline.)

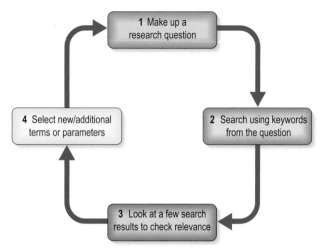

Fig. 17 **Searching for information is an iterative process.**

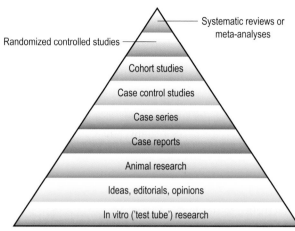

Fig. 20 **Simplified hierarchy of evidence.** (Adapted from SUNY Health Sciences.)

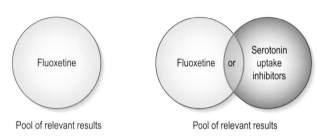

Fig. 18 **Broaden the scope of a search by using synonyms or more general (but still relevant) terms (combine with OR).**

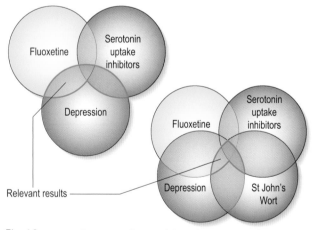

Fig. 19 **Narrow the scope of a search by using more precise terms or by imposing additional required terms (combine with AND).**

Background Extracts of *Hypericum perforatum* (St John's Wort) are widely used to treat depression. Evidence for its efficacy have been criticised on methodological grounds.

Aims To update evidence from randomised trials regarding the effectiveness of *Hypericum* extracts.

Methods We performed a systematic review and meta-analysis of 37 double blind randomised controlled trials that

METHOD

Data sources
We searched for English and non-English language and published and unpublished

RESULTS

Identification of eligible trials
Of 68 possibles, 37 trials met inclusion criteria and contributed 26 comparisons with placebo and 14 comparisons with standard antidepressants (Fig. 1) We then

DISCUSSION

In this updated meta-analysis, we found that *Hypericum perforatum* extracts improved symptoms more than placebo and similarly to standard antidepressants in adults with mild to moderate depression. However, pooled analysis of six recent, large, more precise trials restricted to patients with major depression showed only minimal benefits of *Hypericum* extract compared with placebo

Fig. 21 **Sample journal paper.** (Lende et al 2005).

STOP THINK

- Where do you normally look for information to help make clinical decisions?
- What other sources might you use?
- Think of a therapy for which you would like to find more evidence.
- Create a focused research question that includes patient, intervention, comparison and outcomes.

Sources of further information

Key CAM literature databases

- AMED – Allied and Complementary Medicine Database (fee-based, http://www.bl.uk/collections/health/amed.html). Produced by the British Library. Covers acupuncture, homeopathy, palliative care, Chinese medicine, hospice care, physiotherapy, chiropractic, hypnosis, podiatry, herbalism, occupational therapy, rehabilitation, holistic treatments and osteopathy.
- CHID – Combined Health Information Database (free, http://www.chid.nih.gov/). The CAM section of this database is created by the National Center for Complementary and Alternative Medicine (US government funded) and includes much more than journal articles (newspaper reports, books, bibliographies, etc.) on a wide range of CAM.
- CINAHL – Cumulative Index to Nursing and Allied Health Literature (fee-based, http://www.cinahl.com/). Produced by EBSCO Publishing. Includes journal articles, government reports, dissertations and other publication types. Subject coverage is largely on well-established nursing and allied health disciplines, but with over 35 000 records on CAM topics.
- Cochrane Library (fee-based, http://www.cochrane.org). Produced by the Cochrane Collaboration. The Cochrane are focused on finding high-quality evidence for therapeutic effectiveness, and this is a good place to start looking for the growing number of systematic reviews and controlled trials in CAM. Key sections of the Cochrane library are the Database of Systematic Reviews and the Central Register of Controlled Trials.
- HerbMed (complete access is fee-based though a portion is free, http://www.herbmed.org/). Produced by the Alternative Medicine Foundation. Records for herbs are largely based on PubMed records of articles categorised by areas such as efficacy, activity, safety, and methods of preparation.
- Medline/PubMed (PubMed is free from http://www.pubmed.gov; fee-based Medline access from various providers). Produced by the National Library of Medicine. Medline/PubMed has approximately 100 000 records on CAM therapies, and general searches can be targeted by selecting to limit to the Complementary Medicine subset.
- TRIP – Turning Research Into Practice (fee-based, with some free access, www.tripdatabase.com). This is a federated search tool that searches simultaneously across systematic reviews, guidelines, textbooks, patient leaflets and other publication types. A key advantage of this tool is that the full text is searched, not just titles, so it is easier to find information about CAM buried within, for example, a guideline.

Key CAM resources on the internet

- About Herbs, Botanicals and Other Products (http://www.mskcc.org/mskcc/html/11570.cfm). Produced by the Memorial Sloan-Kettering Cancer Center. A database of herbs and other CAM, providing summary data on constituents, mechanisms, interactions, etc., with references to literature.
- Alternative Medicine Foundation (http://www.amfoundation.org/). This non-profit organisation has a mission of promoting discourse on CAM and providing reliable information to professionals and consumers. The site is notable for its resource guides on CAM modalities and popular health issues.
- Bandolier – Complementary and Alternative Therapies (http://www.jr2.ox.ac.uk/bandolier/booth/booths/altmed.html). Bandolier is an excellent general evidence-based medicine journal, and the section on CAM maintains the high standard of rigorous assessment of evidence for effectiveness.
- Evidence-based Complementary and Alternative Medicine (http://ecam.oxfordjournals.org/).This peer-reviewed, open access journal, from Oxford University Press, has the mission of publishing rigorous scientific research on CAM. It started publication in 2004 and is indexed in PubMed/Medline.
- MedicDirect – Complementary Meds (http://www.medicdirect.co.uk/alt_medicines/). This consumer-oriented site rates therapies according to evidence for effectiveness and presents information about the methods, application, evidence and governing bodies for different modalities.
- National Center for Complementary and Alternative Medicine (http://nccam.nih.gov/). This US government-funded organisation promotes research and public and professional understanding of CAM. The site is notable for its lists of controlled trials and information about conducting trials in CAM.

Assessing evidence for quality and relevance

Marshall F. Dozier and Michael T. Ross

In the previous section ('Finding evidence for CAM'), we described sources of information for CAM and the searching process. Once information has been found, even in peer-reviewed journals, it is necessary to appraise the research findings and evidence for quality and relevance. Appraisal of research methods and results can be time-consuming, so the first step in assessing any evidence from research is to assess whether it is actually relevant to the situation at hand. The formulation of a research question, as described in the previous section, and the identification of research methodologies that yield appropriate data to answer the question, should help in the identification of clear criteria for relevance.

Research methods and CAM

Therapeutic effectiveness of conventional medicine is typically studied using double-blind randomised controlled trials. The aims of this design are to assess whether the treatment has had an effect or whether healing happens regardless of the treatment, and also to reduce the influence of other factors so that the treatment is the only variable being assessed.

Evidence of the effectiveness of interventions is often presented as strong or weak depending on the degree of deviation from the 'gold standard' controlled trial described above. Research methods for evidence have been placed in hierarchies like that shown in Figure 20, with greater importance given to quantitative studies that lend themselves to meta-analysis (the statistical analysis of the results of more than one quantitative study). Many CAM therapies do not permit blinding, which aims to reduce the placebo effect and other influences by requiring either that the patient does not know which intervention they are getting (single blinding) or that neither the patient nor the practitioner knows which intervention is being used (double blinding).

The placebo-controlled double-blind randomised controlled trial is also difficult to implement for some conventional interventions, especially in public health, dental, surgical and psychological contexts. Other methods of gathering empirical evidence for effectiveness are used to study these conventional interventions, and can also be used for CAM. Some examples of study designs which have been used with CAM therapies are presented in Table 9.

Evidence of therapeutic effectiveness is also more complex than the assessment of the efficacy of an intervention. Various questions about effectiveness are presented in Table 10 along with an indication of the type of evidence required to answer the question. For example, risk factors for illness and preventive measures may be investigated using prospective cohort studies, and safety may be investigated using a variety of approaches including randomised controlled trials, cohort studies, surveys and individual case reports (Sackett et al 2000, Lewith et al 2002).

Table 9 **Various study designs use for CAM**

CAM therapy	Study design	Reference
Acupuncture	Randomised controlled trial comparing acupuncture with placebo needles inserted 2 mm deep. Patients and outcome assessors blinded	Ceccherelli F, Rigoni M T, Gagliardi G, Ruzzante L 2002 Comparison of superficial and deep acupuncture in the treatment of lumbar myofascial pain. Clinical Journal of Pain 18(3):149–153
Reflexology	Randomised controlled trial comparing reflexology with basic foot massage. Patients and outcome assessors blinded. Outcomes assessed using rating scales and semi-structured interviews	Ross C S, Hamilton J, Macrae G, Docherty C, Gould A, Cornbleet M A 2002 A pilot study to evaluate the effect of reflexology on mood and symptom rating of advanced cancer patients. Palliative Medicine 16(6):544–545
Nutrition/diet	Multicentre case-control study	Jain M G, Hislop G T, Howe G R, Ghadirian P 1999 Plant foods, antioxidants and prostate cancer risk: findings from case-control studies in Canada. Nutrition and Cancer 34(2):173–184

Table 10 **Questions to ask when evaluating CAM (Spencer & Jacobs 1999)**

Types of evidence	Validation questions
Experimental evidence	Is the practice efficacious when examined experimentally?
Clinical (practice) evidence	Is the practice effective when applied clinically?
Safety evidence	Is the practice safe?
Comparative evidence	Is it the best practice for the problem?
Summary evidence	Is the practice known and evaluated?
Rational evidence	Is the practice rational, progressing, and contributing to medical and scientific understanding?
Demand evidence	Do consumers and practitioners want the practice?
Satisfaction evidence	Is it meeting the expectations of patients and practitioners?
Cost evidence	Is the practice inexpensive to operate and/or cost-effective? Is it provided by payers?
Meaning evidence	Is the practice the right one for the individual?

Appraisal of information from websites

Information on the internet presents a particular challenge, since quality control, if any, is exercised by the creators of websites. Research has shown that although there are high-quality websites discussing or promoting CAM, a proportion of websites give misleading and even harmful information (Schmidt & Ernst 2004).

What to look for in assessing websites for quality of information:

■ Authority – what qualifications does the author of the website have, and are the qualifications relevant to the subject covered? Does the author give complete contact information?
■ Currency – how recently was the website updated, or is there even a date? How recent is any cited reference?
■ Evidence base – is the information accurate? Are there any references to research that supports the claims made on the site? Does the site report evidence both for and against the therapy? Are the cited references readily available? Do they actually support the claims made on the site?
■ Sponsorship – where is the website hosted (e.g. is it private, or part of a commercial or non-profit organisation)? Is there any advertising or sponsorship on the site? Who funded the research that is cited to support the site's claims? What interest might the host, advertisers or funding bodies have in the claims made on the site?

Appraisal of the professional literature

Critical appraisal even of peer-reviewed journal articles requires just as much attention as a website. Here are questions to consider when reading a report of a qualitative study, quantitative study or review:

■ Are the aims of the study clear? If the objectives of the study are not clear, or if they are not relevant to the searcher's research question, then it is not worth reading the article.
■ Did the authors use an appropriate research method for issue in question? It is helpful to think about what kind of data will help to fill the information gap identified by the authors, and how that data might best be measured and collected.

- Are the research methods rigorous? In the description of the methods, is it possible to see that the requirements of the study design were met? For example, in a blinded trial, what was the mechanism for blinding, and would it have been possible to circumvent it?
- Do the measured results actually address the objectives of the study? Sometimes researchers get distracted from their initial objectives, and sometimes pains are taken to interpret the results in a way that fits an early hypothesis. It is worth comparing the 'results' section with the 'conclusions' section to make sure they are consistent.
- Are the conclusions reached in the study relevant to the local situation? Was the study population big enough? Is the patient or population(s) described in the paper similar to the local population? Are the interventions described available locally?

Brief appraisal of a sample paper

The sample journal paper (see Fig. 21) gives a reference to a systematic literature review on the effectiveness of St John's wort for depression.

In appraising this example reference, the key elements to examine are the aims, methods, results and conclusions, which should be described in enough detail to be reproducible. The aim of this review was 'To update evidence from randomised trials regarding the effectiveness of *Hypericum* [St John's wort] extracts.' This aim does match the research question we formulated, though we need to dig a little deeper into the paper to find out if it compares St John's wort with serotonin uptake inhibitors. Herbal remedies, like conventional medications, do lend themselves well to the randomised controlled trial, so the selection of this study design is appropriate.

The methods used in such a literature review should lead to the discovery of all comparable randomised controlled trials. In this case the reviewers searched in the Cochrane controlled trials register and in PubMed, as well as building on previous, undescribed searches, so it might be commented that they used limited data sources.

Criteria for inclusion and exclusion should be explicit and should ensure an unbiased and consistent selection of relevant papers for the review. In this paper, the reviewers list the criteria for study design, participants, experimental and control interventions and outcome measures. The other

STOP THINK In designing an approach to finding evidence of therapeutic effectiveness, deciding on the type of research design giving the right data for analysis is a similar process to designing an original study. If you were designing an experiment on the effectiveness of massage therapy:
- Which condition would you select for treatment in the study?
- What type of massage would you use?
- How would you measure the effects of the therapy?
- What variables might you need to account for?

methods (data extraction and statistical analysis) are described to a similar level of detail.

The results describe both the results of the literature review, and at a deeper level, the methods and results of the trials. Analyses of the methods and results of the trials are clearly presented in text, tables and figures, with confidence intervals. Studies were classed for comparison and meta-analysis by type of depression, trial size and control (placebo or conventional antidepressants).

The discussion gives a measured presentation of factors that must be borne in mind in looking at the results, including problems with publication bias, variations in rigour of research methodology, variables in study groups. Conclusions match the results and state that there is little benefit or no difference compared to placebo in mild to moderate depression, and no difference compared to standard antidepressants.

Summary

Appraisal of evidence for use of CAM should and can be as rigorous as that of conventional therapies. Appraisal should be based on the type of information presented and according to research design.

The literature and evidence base for CAM is evolving rapidly. However, it is common for the conclusions in systematic reviews of therapeutic effectiveness of even conventional interventions to indicate that there is not enough evidence or only poor quality evidence on which to draw. There is a healthy debate on tackling the complexities of research and evidence-based practice in CAM (Lewith et al 2002, Kane 2004).

Sources of further information

Sources of detailed guidance on assessing the quality of health-related websites
- BIOME: http://biome.ac.uk/
- Health on the Net: http://www.hon.ch/
- Judge: websites for health: http://www.judgehealth.org.uk/

Sources of detailed guidance on critical appraisal of journal articles
- Critical Appraisal Skills Programme: http://www.phru.nhs.uk/casp/
- Greenhalgh T 2006 How to read a paper: the basics of evidence based medicine, 3rd edn. Blackwell, Malden, MA
- Scottish Intercollegiate Guidelines Network: http://www.sign.ac.uk/

Research methods in CAM
- Kane M 2004 Research made easy in complementary and alternative medicine. Churchill Livingstone, Edinburgh
- Lewith G, Jonas W B, Walach H 2002 Clinical research in complementary therapies: principles, problems and solutions. Churchill Livingstone, Edinburgh
- Nahin R, Straus S 2001 Research into complementary and alternative medicine: problems and potential. British Medical Journal 322:161–164
- Pocock S J 1983 Clinical trials: a practical approach. Wiley & Sons, Chichester

Users' perspective on CAM

Trends and perceptions

David Brown and Mike Porter

Many of the disciplines of complementary and alternative medicine (CAM), such as herbalism and acupuncture, were the conventional medicine of the past. These were the treatments of choice, familiar, obtainable within the community, part of the local culture. Their role has been usurped by what we now call conventional medicine, a product of technological advances which have permitted improved diagnostic procedures, modern pharmacology and surgical techniques. Diseases such as poliomyelitis, tuberculosis and smallpox have, in the Western world, been virtually eradicated. The morbidity and premature mortality associated with diabetes, ischaemic heart disease and asthma have been dramatically reduced. Why then is there a significant and increasing move back to CAM by consumers throughout the Western world?

Current situation

In the UK, the National Health Service costs £74 billion per year, of which £10 billion is spent on drugs. Consumers also spend £10 billion annually on the purchase of medicines and private care. Figure 22 illustrates the range of CAM therapies available at one private health spa. It is estimated that £1.6 billion is spent annually on CAM in the UK. Surveys have shown that 20% of respondents have used CAM in the preceding year and 14% have consulted a CAM practitioner (Ernst 2000).

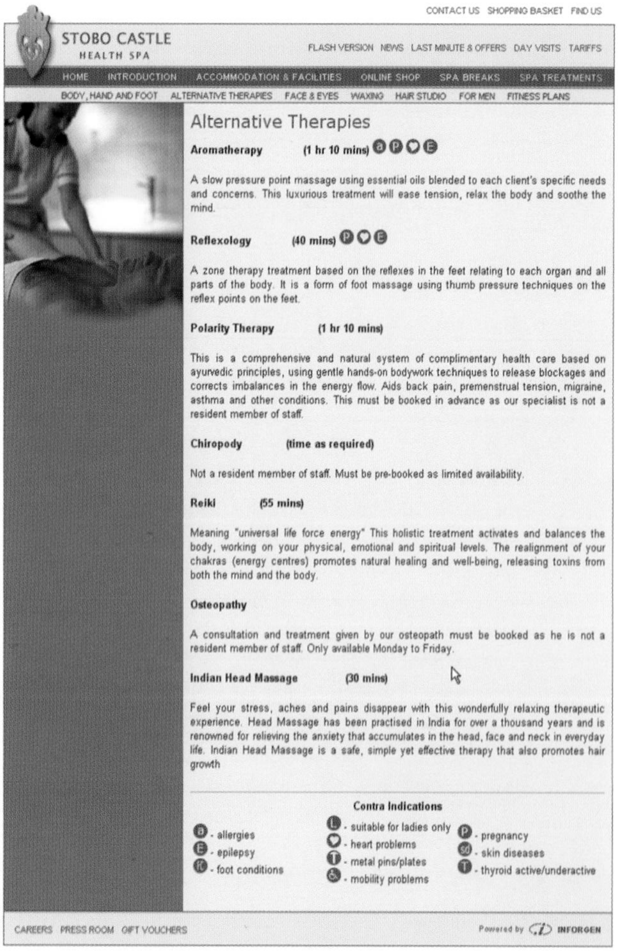

According to evidence given by the Royal Pharmaceutical Society to the House of Lords Select Committee on Science and Technology (2000), this is a growing trend, as indicated by a 50% increase in sales of herbal products between 1994 and 1998.

A survey in England found that the most commonly consulted CAM therapists were osteopaths, chiropractors, aromatherapists, reflexologists and acupuncturists (Thomas et al 2001).

Compared to other Western countries, the UK is not a big user of CAM. Over 60% of Germans have used CAM in the preceding year (Fig. 23). Growth in use is indicated also by the Canadian National Population Health Study (NPHS), which recorded an increase from 15% to 19% in adults consulting an alternative practitioner between 1994 and 1998.

Who uses CAM?

The Canadian NPHS (1994) is typical in showing a female preponderance of 4:3 in CAM use except for chiropractic, used equally by both sexes. Middle-aged people use CAM more, as do the relatively affluent and well educated. Those with chronic conditions and chronic pain also tend to make more use of CAM.

Patterns of use of CAM and conventional care

It is clear that people do not use CAM exclusively but will also use conventional medicine for specific types of complaint and for specific purposes. CAM users are more

Fig. 22 **CAM therapies are often available at health spas throughout the UK.** (Courtesy of Stobo Castle Health Spa, Scotland).

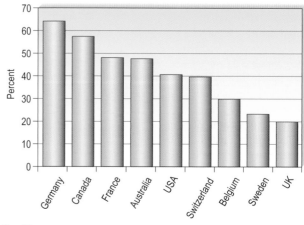

Fig. 23 **Prevalence of CAM use** (Ernst 2000).

likely than non-users to have seen a medical specialist, had their blood pressure checked and consulted their primary physician over 10 times in the preceding year (NPHS 1994).

Users' perception of healthcare

The initial step in obtaining healthcare is to seek a consultation. CAM users may prefer not to use conventional care, perceiving it as rushed, impersonal and interested only in the pathology, not the whole person.

The average consultation time in general practice in the UK is 10 minutes. Waiting times for secondary care in the UK are increasingly long, defined in months rather than weeks. Although there is no clear relationship between waiting times and use of CAM, patients may opt for a treatment system where they feel more in control.

A CAM practitioner is easily accessible, provided one has the financial resources, and may spend up to an hour with a patient, enquiring not only about the specific problem but also about their lifestyle, their diet and their attitudes, building up an empathic relationship. The patient has the opportunity to interact with the therapist, to feel listened to and to feel valued. Such an approach significantly increases the chances of any treatment being felt to be successful.

In the UK, the NHS provides free care. This is predominantly conventional, with limited access to homeopathy, hypnotherapy and acupuncture. Unless obtained through the NHS, the patient will have to pay for CAM treatment. This might be seen as a disincentive to using CAM but, conversely, is thought to increase the patient's 'investment' in the treatment and an increased determination to perceive that treatment as beneficial.

Elsewhere, especially in the US and in Europe, healthcare costs are paid by the patient or by their insurers. The latter are increasingly willing either to fund CAM treatment options or to encourage patients to use them to self-treat. In Germany, the decision to be treated by conventional or complementary therapies is less 'black and white'. Most German physicians are trained in naturopathic treatment and all pharmacists are taught herbal medicine. Thus a patient can receive both types of therapy through the same treatment pathway. When surveyed, most Germans expressed a preference to be treated by a physician who also had training in complementary medicine (Pascoe 2002).

Patients regard themselves as consumers and wish to exercise choice over healthcare as much as they do over other purchases. If conventional care does not correspond to their value judgements and attitudes, then an alternative will be sought which seems more empathic.

Conventional care may be perceived as authoritarian; doctors are traditionally regarded as socially superior and omniscient, unused to having their opinion queried. Medical 'gatekeepers', preventing direct patient access to their chosen diagnostic or treatment option, control access to treatment. Modern, affluent patients have the education and the resources to seek out their own information and the confidence to question authority.

CAM treatments appeal to their users as being natural, steeped in tradition, and holistic. They are considered safe and their provision is often in a pleasant and relaxed environment. Although they may not have scientific explanation, patients may find the explanation of their efficacy intuitively acceptable and concordant with their own beliefs that reject modern technology, science and the establishment. They may feel if one particular therapy does not work then no harm is done and they can move on to another.

Patient studies have indicated a high level of satisfaction with CAM, not only in the quality of the experience in terms of time spent and therapist empathy, but also in treatment efficacy (Resch et al 1997).

Conventional treatment is seen as 'high tech, low touch' as opposed to 'low tech, high touch'. It can be unpleasant, have side effects and dangers and can be perceived as treating the disease, not the patient.

We have been led to expect a long and healthy life, free from the risk of premature death and debility. As a result of living longer, we become exposed to the diseases of old age, cancer, heart disease and diabetes. Conventional medicine has developed to deal with such problems.

We also have an expectation of a positive sense of well-being, not simply an absence of disease. As a result of the pressures and the pace of modern life, we are exposed to the problems of obesity, overindulgence in alcohol, anxiety, low mood and chronic fatigue. These are problems which we expect, in vain, conventional care to help deal with. Conventional care has offered technological 'cures' such as benzodiazepines, which proved to cause more problems than solutions. Thus let down, we turn to the alternative sector who, in return for a portion of our new affluence, will listen, empathise and offer hope.

Conventional care has the advantage for patients of a diagnostic process. CAM practitioners are not able to offer patients the reassurance of a precise label for their illness and the exclusion of serious possibilities supported by diagnostic tools like CT scan, MRI, biopsy reports etc. On the other hand, parents whose child has been diagnosed with Down's syndrome report that they turn to CAM therapists for a more positive and supportive interpretation of their child's prospects than that received from the doctors who make the diagnosis. Sophisticated CAM users may, then, consult conventional medicine for a diagnosis before turning to CAM for their preferred form of treatment. A Canadian population study showed that 7% of those given a conventional prescription by a physician substituted a natural health product (NPHS 1998). Consumers may also appreciate that if conventional care fails to provide a cure, CAM may at least provide symptomatic relief without the side effects and risks.

Others may consult a CAM practitioner when conventional medicine fails to provide a diagnosis or to offer treatment for their condition. Patients may feel rejected, or even that they are perceived as fraudulent, by conventional care in this situation.

In conclusion, a person making the choice to use CAM and/or conventional medicine may look at the positive and negative attributes of each. These are summarised in Table 11.

- Why do patients use CAM?
- How do patients get reliable CAM information?
- What role does the healthcare professional have to ensure patients get objective information on CAM therapies?

Table 11 **Users' perspective**		
	CAM	**Conventional medicine**
Positive attributes	Patient centred	Evidence-based practice
	Empathic	Scientifically based efficacy
	'Natural'	Free
	Few adverse effects	
	Pleasant experience	
	Accessible	
	Non-establishment	
	Efficacy based on personal experience/testimony	
Negative attributes	Lack of objective scientific evidence	Establishment
	Cost	Disease oriented
		Limited treatment options
		Lack of time
		Waiting lists
		Adverse effects of treatment

Sources of further information

- Health Canada: www.hc-sc.gc.ca/
- National Center for Complementary and Alternative Medicine: http://nccam.nih.gov
- NHS Direct Online: www.nhsdirect.nhs.uk

Users' sources of CAM information

David Brown and Mike Porter

CAM users, as much as professionals, should be able to source reliable data. When seeking information, people turn increasingly to the internet (Figs 24 and 25). Various studies have shown that between 36% and 55% of all internet users have accessed medical information. Over 40% of breast cancer patients in both Canada and the US used the internet to investigate their illness and its treatment (Satterlund et al 2003). In an American study in 2001, 48% of those seeking information on alternative medicine searched the internet (Baker et al 2003).

Search engines most readily direct the consumer to sites that provide unsubstantiated and unreferenced claims for CAM products as well as offering them for sale. They often do not provide any indication of the quality of the information available on the site. Lay users may also have a problem with 'information literacy', the capacity to understand and interpret the scientific and statistical basis of the information provided. Serious doubts have been expressed about the safety of such information, particularly in the area of cancer treatments where not only are unsubstantiated treatments promoted but patients can be advised against conventional treatments (Schmidt & Ernst 2004).

Information online from academic journals in the form of evidence-based articles is less prominent and less accessible for lay users.

It therefore may be difficult for the consumer to obtain unbiased information. However, this appears to be changing internationally. In the UK, the Consumers' Association's *Health Which?* magazine aims to provide information to allow the layman to make an informed decision.

The House of Lords report on CAM (2000) concluded that the ideal repository of such information should be the NHS Direct Online website. Some information is now available through this website.

In the US, the National Center for Complementary and Alternative Medicine (NCCAM) publishes the results of its studies on its website and in Canada, the Health Canada website has extensive information.

It is hoped that one benefit of the move to incorporate CAM practitioners in legally regulated bodies will be the provision of objective information about these therapies (see Section 2).

Consumers' attitudes may also be led by the media. Information on CAM is widely available in newspapers, magazines and television. Currently the media appear to favour CAM therapies, with CAM options often receiving uncritical support in lifestyle articles and products being advertised widely in newspapers and magazines.

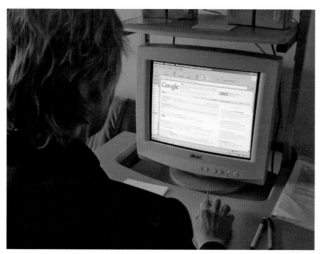

Fig. 24 **A patient searching on the internet at home for information on homeopathy.** (Reproduced with permission of Google, Inc.)

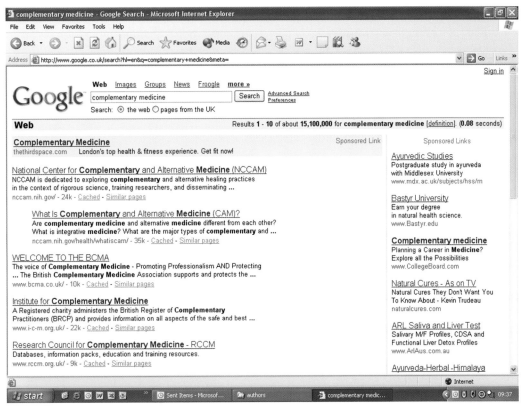

Fig. 25 **Google search on 'complementary medicine' brings up more than 15 million hits.** (Reproduced with permission of Google, Inc.)

An important motivator to using CAM is word-of-mouth testimonial from other users and self-help groups. Belief in the power of CAM is often an 'act of faith' rather than an acceptance of fact based on scientific evidence. Consequently those who have experienced benefit and relief of symptoms at the hands of a CAM practitioner are liable to be enthusiastic proponents, contrasting the benefits of this treatment favourably with the failure of conventional care.

For the patient who is contemplating using a CAM therapy, the WHO (2002) has produced guidelines that identify questions which should be addressed (Table 12).

Patients should expect to be able to obtain objective information about CAM from their conventional physician. As CAM has not, until recently, been taught in the medical curriculum, they may not get advice that is informed or objective. Patients may also be reluctant to ask conventional doctors for advice on CAM because they perceive the conventional practitioners disapprove. In a study in the US, it was found that 72% of those using CAM would not tell their physician (Kaye et al 2000).

Consumers' attitude to evidence

It can be difficult to be objective about one's own illness or health concerns. Particularly in the areas where CAM is used, it is possible that the 'placebo effect' plays a large part in any perceived benefit. Individuals may reject the suggestion that their improved well-being is as a result of such an effect and, equally, prefer not to explore the objective evidence for a treatment. Conversely, if a therapy produces benefits, even through a placebo effect, then many would consider this worthwhile.

Consumer studies have shown that there is a desire for information that is accessible, credible and authoritative (Baker 2003). Many understand that the information available is often unreliable and bemoan the failure of government organisations to provide guidance for the use of CAM.

Table 12 **Questions for CAM users (WHO 2002)**
■ Is it safe?
■ Is it suitable for someone with my condition?
■ Does it have the potential to prevent or improve symptoms, and contribute to health and well-being?
■ Is the therapy provided by a qualified (and preferably registered) practitioner with adequate training, skills and knowledge?
■ Are any medicinal products and materials used of assured quality?
■ Is the treatment method acceptable?
■ Is the CAM available and accessible?
■ How long will the course of therapy last?
■ What will it cost?

- Prostatic cancer is the most common cancer in men in the UK.
- Men are more likely to die WITH prostatic cancer than FROM it.
- Watchful waiting gives an 80% 10-year survival in localised prostatic cancer and 30% for poorly differentiated cancers.
- Watchful waiting gives the same survival as radical surgery in localised prostatic cancer, with a lower incidence of side effects from intervention.
- After radical prostatectomy, up to 70% of men are impotent and up to 20% incontinent.

Source: Cancer Research UK 2002.

Recipients of healthcare increasingly regard themselves as 'consumers' or 'users' as their need and capacity to participate in decision-making increases. They are no longer willing to assume a passive role, relying on the wisdom and beneficence of their healthcare provider. They need to be able to access objective information about conventional and alternative medicine to enable them to make an informed choice. Treatment must also conform to their belief systems.

Healthcare providers in the conventional sector must recognise this change and accept it as a positive step, embracing and learning from all that is positive in CAM.

Case study

Qualitative study

In a study of twenty-nine Canadian men (mean age 65) diagnosed with prostate cancer, it was reported that only one-third had used CAM therapies prior to diagnosis, but that two-thirds had used CAM subsequently. All men reported that the diagnosis of prostate cancer had instilled feelings of fear and loss of control in their lives, both of which affected their decisions about both conventional and CAM therapies, over time.

The study reported that most men who used CAM therapies were 'pushed' into its use as a result of conventional medicine not meeting their beliefs and expectations. These men were more likely to access CAM therapies when they felt that conventional treatment options were limited. They were further pushed towards CAM because they held relatively strong beliefs about the risks of adverse side effects of conventional treatments, and 'pulled' towards CAM as they held relatively weak beliefs about the adverse side effects of CAM therapies.

> Not only does the prostatectomy have a fairly high morbidity/side effects, but what really clinched it for me was when I read that in 10% to 40% of cases of men that have radical prostatectomy, they also have recurrence, so they really have the worst of all worlds in my view which is to possibly be incontinent and impotent, but at the same time still have cancer.

Furthermore, rather than just 'wait and see', many men preferred to do something and sought out CAM therapies that suited them, which also gave them a sense of being in control.

> So, my conclusion is nobody knows, it's a crapshoot ... I'd rather take a little bit of charge and control of myself.

> Watchful waiting is a tricky business ... why wait for clear signs, why not do something anyway.

Some of these men were further pushed towards CAM use by negative experiences of conventional practitioners:

> Look at the example of my urologist ... I wanted to talk to him about me ... about the operation. When he found out I wasn't going to have the operation, he was no longer interested in talking to me at all. I was in his way. I was taking up space and taking up time ... .

Quantitative study

Of 534 Canadian men diagnosed with prostate cancer (mean age 69), 22% reported using CAM prior to diagnosis and 30% using CAM post-diagnosis. The study found that the main explanatory factors for CAM use were:
- attendance at a support group
- conventional hormonal treatment (associated with more serious illness)
- stronger beliefs in the efficacy and low risks of side effects of CAM therapies.

Sources: Boon et al (2003a, 2003b).

A personal experience

Allan D. Cumming

Case study

The twinges in my back have been troublesome for a few days. But as I bend over in the shower to rinse my hair, it goes. Suddenly, standing up straight is agony, and even a Quasimodo-like hunch brings tears to the eyes. Wonderful timing: Saturday morning, on holiday in a small seaside town, due on the first tee in an hour for an important golf game, struck down by a severe, acute disability. Even my physician-level knowledge of orthopaedics leads to a diagnosis of prolapsed intervertebral disc.

First reflex: give me drugs. I don't know what proportion of the population carry ibuprofen around with them, but since the first skeletal creaks arrived in my 40s I have capsules, tablets, liquid, gels, whatever Tesco and Boots between them can come up with. Ten minutes after two rapid-action liquid-filled capsules and a generous lumbar application of gel, the pain eases slightly. Maybe it would have anyway. But at least I can move.

Next – more drugs. Anadin Extra – paracetamol and aspirin in combination. Two of those make no discernible difference. Still cannot stand straight, and walking an excruciating effort. Not even sure if I can drive a car, and certainly not a golf ball. OK – cancel golf, drink tea, and consider the options. Clearly I need expert help.

Case study–cont'd

Option 1. Go to the hospital accident and emergency department. The nearest is 30 miles away – a long taxi ride. Visions of waiting for hours to be seen by a neophyte and being sent away with more ibuprofen. Or even worse – an emergency MRI scan, urgent discectomy, weeks of convalescence, dressings, bedpans, catheters, drips, needles, MRSA, necrotising fasciitis … .

Option 2. Consult local general practitioner. It is Saturday morning. Phone call indicates that cover is by a regional GP service, based in the same town as the accident and emergency department. Difficult to see what the doctor would do other than send me there anyway with more ibuprofen. It all seems a bit pointless, I need some treatment, something to make me better, but preferably without scalpels and wounds … .

Option 3. The Yellow Pages. I am amazed to see that an osteopath is practising just 400 yards up the road, one of two in the town. In the advertisement his name is followed by a veritable cascade of letters … impressive; however, I have no idea what any of them mean. The advertisement describes 'Gentle soft tissue massage techniques, stretching and manipulation to relieve muscle tension, pain and stiffness in the body.' It all seems a little soft-touch considering the depths of my distress, but what is there to lose. I call at 10.15 a.m. He has a patient till 11 but can see me immediately after that. I struggle into socks and shoes and commence a Parkinson's-like shuffle in his direction. After 15 painful and undignified minutes I arrive outside a handsome villa in a quiet street. An elderly lady is being helped into her car. She still looks pretty bent and stiff, but is smiling.

After a waiting time of 10 minutes I am greeted by John, an instantly likeable man in his 40s, dressed informally in shirt and chinos. I am ushered into a plush, bookcase lined consulting room. Once seated, there is a notice with a scale of fees facing me: £35 for the first consultation. At that moment I would happily have paid three times that for any chance of relief.

After some classically open questions, John begins to gather a systematic history which even I can recognise from orthopaedic attachments at medical school. Presenting complaint, presence or absence of bladder or bowel disturbance (none so far), past history, family history, social history … a familiar catechism. It all takes an age and I eye the treatment table longingly.

Eventually I am positioned on the couch (Fig. 26). After some classical straight-leg raising (or lack of it) the osteopathy begins. I am on my side, facing the bookcase, as the gentle probing of my lumbar regions proceeds. I recognise some well-kent titles – *Macleod's Textbook of Clinical Examination, Davidson's Textbook of Medicine,* several anatomy books – beside the less 'conventional' volumes. I am vaguely aware of three things – the treatment has not actually been explained to me; I have not been asked to consent to it or sign anything; and I have not been told what might or might not be wrong with me. Just at that moment, however, none of this seems very important.

The pressure of the massage is gradually increased and settles to a regular rhythm of what I am told is 'cross-fibre work'. It is not painful in itself, and perhaps the pre-existing discomfort is easing – I am not sure. It goes on for 15 minutes. Then I am warned of some impending 'gentle manipulation'. Various extremities are grasped firmly and used to exert a strong, sudden stretch force on my spine. It is not the kind of vicious, snapping technique that I mentally associate with chiropractic, but vigorous none the less. A few more minutes of cross-fibre work round off the session.

The moment of truth – getting off the couch. Gingerly I weight-bear. There is still pain, but definitely less than before … and … I can stand upright! Hallelujah! A brisk perambulation around the room is completed in style. I am happy. I am grateful. John suggests a follow-up session 2 days later. I gladly agree. We shake hands. I go out into the sunshine, and anyone who had seen me arrive would surely have been impressed. Not exactly skipping, but undoubtedly mobile.

So, in a wholly unrandomised, unblinded and uncontrolled trial where $n=1$ with 0 degrees of freedom, did osteopathy work? Well, like the curate's egg, in parts. It did not offer diagnosis or prognosis. It did not cure. But it did give relief, and a standard of personal service that puts the NHS to shame. Would I go back? Absolutely. Do I think it should be provided free by the NHS? – well yes I do, it seems wrong that only people with £35 to spend should receive the relief it offers. But I can't help thinking that John seems to be doing pretty well as it is, even with what must be a fairly small catchment area, and that perhaps a 6-month waiting list and a Health Board on his back is not what he – or his patients – are after. At the very least we would all have to fill in many, many more forms. Perhaps things are best as they are. It is good to know that he is there should I need him again.

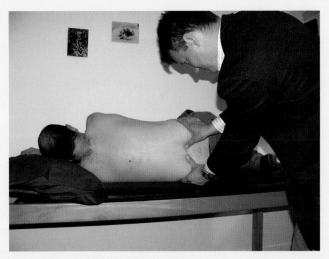

Fig. 26 **On the couch at the osteopath's.**

Communication and relationships in CAM

History taking and giving advice

Kirsty J. Boyd and Bryan Allan

Complementary and alternative therapies are here to stay. Increasing numbers of patients are using them and seeking information about them. How can CAM be integrated safely into conventional medicine? Doctors need to understand, and be able to explain to their patients, the risks and benefits of a range of therapies. Good doctor–patient relationships, which balance patient and doctor perspectives in a dialogue about the best way to address the patient's problems, are a prerequisite for this (Fig. 27). Doctors must also know how to communicate and work effectively with CAM therapists.

History taking

Why did you not tell me you were using CAM?

Although more patients than ever are using complementary therapies, they often fail to tell their doctors about it (Fig. 28). Patients describe several barriers to open disclosure: failure to ask or ignoring patient cues, opposition to CAM use by doctors along with their emphasis on a scientific evidence base for treatments, anticipation of a negative response from the doctor, a belief that the doctor will be unable or unwilling to contribute useful information, and the perception that CAM use is not relevant to a conventional consultation or treatment plan. Doctors who are open-minded, willing to listen and honest about the limitations of their own knowledge about CAM are appreciated. Patients often want their doctor to be aware of their CAM use and to provide advice about it (Adler & Fosket 1999, Rao et al 1999, Schofield et al 2003).

Doctors can be reluctant to initiate a discussion about CAM for various reasons. Lack of knowledge and confidence in offering information may be compounded by beliefs that much or all CAM is outside the biomedical remit, and potentially harmful. When the patient has a life-limiting illness such as cancer, the doctor may fear that a discussion about CAM will open up difficult issues such as the meaning of the illness, coping strategies, and the patient's emotional or existential concerns about their future (Tasaki et al 2002, Zollman & Vickers 1999c). Education in CAM for health professionals must address communication issues.

No assumptions should be made about which patient is likely to be using CAM and an enquiry should always be made about it. Disclosure will be facilitated if history taking proceeds in a patient-centred manner, listening to patients' accounts of their problems, and eliciting their ideas, concerns and expectations in the context of building up a relationship with them. Relating to patients as people and showing respect for their views will enable the doctor to explore potentially sensitive areas such as CAM use successfully. This forms the basis of effective dialogue about the contribution of such treatments to care, and ensures that any safety issues are identified and addressed (Table 13).

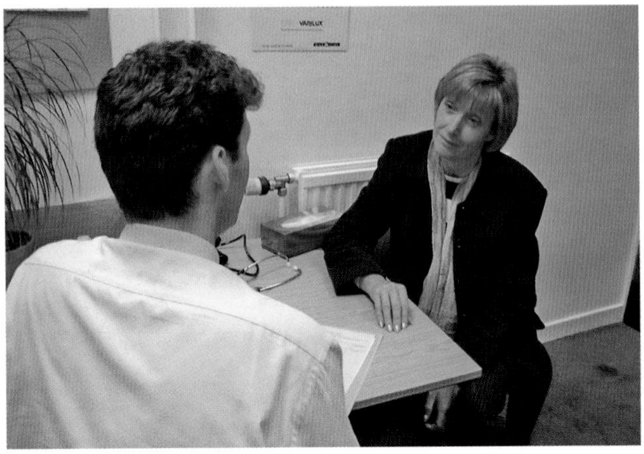

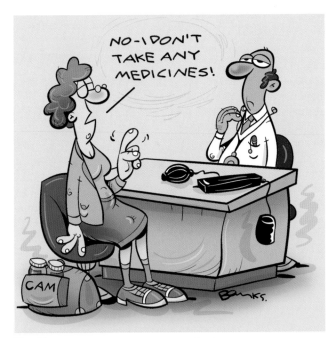

Fig. 28 **'No I don't take any regular medications.'**

Fig. 27 **Consulting the doctor.**

Table 13 **Useful questions to ask patients (Zollman & Vickers 1999b)**
Behaviour
■ Have you tried any other treatment approaches for this problem?
■ Have you ever seen a complementary or alternative medicine practitioner about this problem?
■ Have you ever tried changing your diet because you thought it might help?
■ Have you used any herbal or natural remedies bought from a chemist, pharmacy or health food shop?
Attitudes
■ What are you hoping to gain from your complementary treatment?
■ What encouraged you to try complementary medicine?
Collaboration
■ Would you ask your complementary therapist to keep me informed about your treatment and progress?

Explanation and advice

Patients choose to seek help from CAM for many reasons so any discussion with their doctor about the role of such therapy in their overall care should start by exploring the understanding and expectations of the patient (and informal carer).

There is a common contradiction in patients' views of the safety of complementary medicines. Complementary medicines are assumed to be safe because they are not pharmaceutical products. Patients may be unaware that certain over-the-counter herbal medicines have potentially serious adverse effects including liver and kidney failure, and some produce significant interactions with conventional medications (Giveon et al 2004). Conventional medicines are subject to strict testing before marketing and post-marketing surveillance. However, withdrawal of a drug due to adverse effects is much more likely to attract media attention, which can compound the view that prescribed medication is potentially unsafe. Information about complementary therapies is often obtained from the media, family and friends or the internet. A review of websites on complementary and alternative medicine for cancer found that the information was of very variable quality. Many sites endorsed unproven therapies, some of which were likely to be harmful (Schmidt & Ernst 2004). There is a clear need for patients to be able to access balanced advice from their doctor which takes account of their values and perspectives. Doctors must also ensure that the patient does not have a life-threatening illness requiring urgent treatment, an illness for which conventional medicine has clear and effective treatment (e.g. diabetes, hypothyroidism, anaemia, parasitic infections) or needs further investigation to establish the cause of the symptoms.

The 'typical' CAM user tends to be well educated, to appreciate a person-centred approach to care, and to have reduced health status due to a chronic or life-threatening condition such as cancer, HIV-related illnesses, chronic pain, anxiety or depression or a medically unexplained illness. Complementary therapies may be sought as an adjunct or replacement for conventional treatment considered insufficient to address the person's problems fully. CAM may be perceived as a way of making an active

Table 14 **Shared decision-making**
■ Explore patient (and family) experiences and expectations of CAM and conventional treatments.
■ Elicit reasons for CAM use.
■ Build a partnership through dialogue and respect for the patient's views.
■ Exchange and discuss information and evidence about treatments for the patient's condition; balance benefits with risks/side effects, and consider uncertainties.
■ Offer recommendations based on patient preferences, and review options.
■ Agree care plan and follow-up arrangements.

contribution to well-being and increasing the chance of a positive outcome, or be an important aspect of maintaining hope (Rao et al 1999, Mackenzie et al 1999, Schofield et al 2003, George et al 2004).

Having elicited the patient's reasons for using or considering CAM and their experiences and expectations, the doctor can take account of this when exchanging information about the patient's condition and treatment options. Benefits, risks and uncertainties about possible CAM and conventional treatments can be considered. The doctor will then be able to offer recommendations based on a full understanding of the patient's preferences, and advise about the risks of making changes to current treatment without consulting their doctor. Finally a care plan and clear follow-up arrangements should be negotiated (Frenkel & Borkan 2003, Zollman & Vickers 1999c).

Table 14 identifies the shared decision-making process between the conventional doctor and patient.

When CAM is first discussed, and at subsequent reviews, it is important for the doctor to screen for undiagnosed illnesses and any physical or medication-related adverse effects. Potential psychological problems should also be considered. A potential danger of empowering patients to play an active part in improving their health is that they come to believe that they are solely responsible for the outcome. Others may accede to pressure from family or friends to use CAM while having little confidence in it. Denial can sometimes be a helpful, temporary coping strategy but if it persists, and leads to inappropriate behaviour such as seeking relief through repeated CAM treatments without evidence of psychological adjustment to the condition, it should be addressed (Zollman & Vickers 1999c).

Organising care and teamwork

Kirsty J. Boyd and Bryan Allan

Should a doctor refer or delegate to a CAM therapist?

Patients generally access CAM by self-referral, referral by a doctor (usually their general practitioner), or may receive treatment from their own doctor or a therapist working in that practice. What are the legal and ethical obligations of doctors in these situations?

A doctor who does not feel able to advise a patient about complementary therapies may not wish to refer or delegate

care. They should make it clear that they will respect the patient's choice, and seek to maintain a continuing professional relationship with that patient (BMA 1999). An important aspect of the doctor's duty of care is to advise patients of all the available options for treatment of their condition. As some forms of CAM (such as acupuncture) become more evidence-based, regulated and accepted, doctors need to consider the extent to which they are obliged to provide patients with information about such therapies (Weir 2003). They may wish to use a simple

Table 15 CAM checklist for doctors considering referral of patients

- Is the CAM therapy safe and supported by some evidence of effectiveness?
- Is the therapist registered with a professional organisation?
- Does this organisation have a register accessible to the public?
- Does it have a code of practice covering:
  Standards and competencies for its practitioners?
  Contraindications and limits of competence?
  Relationships and communication between therapist, patient, and other health professionals?
  Record keeping?
- Does the regulatory body have effective disciplinary procedures and sanctions?
- Is there a clear complaints mechanism?
- What qualifications does the therapist hold?
- What is the length and quality of training?
- How long has the therapist been practising?
- Is the therapist covered by professional indemnity insurance?

checklist to evaluate a particular CAM therapy service (Table 15).

If a CAM treatment is available under the NHS (e.g. NHS homeopathic hospitals and clinics, and some osteopathy clinics), the general practitioner can refer a patient in the normal way. It is important, however, to be clear about the distinction between referral and delegation (GMC 2001, Zollman & Vickers 1999a).

Referral

Referral involves transferring some or all of a doctor's responsibility for the patient's care; usually on a temporary basis and for a particular purpose that falls outside the doctor's competence. If referral is not to another medical practitioner, the doctor has to ensure that the healthcare professional is accountable to a statutory regulatory body. A doctor, usually the general practitioner, retains overall responsibility for the patient's management. This means that doctors can refer patients to complementary therapists who are registered healthcare professionals (e.g. doctors, nurses, allied health professionals) or such professionals offering CAM as a supplement to their normal services. Similarly, referrals can be made to practitioners in osteopathy and chiropractic who are registered with the relevant statutory regulatory bodies, so fully accountable to that body for their actions. The referring doctor must be satisfied that the patient will benefit from the type of treatment involved, but is not responsible for the detail of the treatment given (BMA 1999, Zollman & Vickers 1999a).

Delegation

Delegation occurs when a doctor asks a student or healthcare professional to carry out a treatment or procedure on their behalf. Enough information about the patient and the treatment needed has to be passed on, and the doctor remains responsible for the patient's management. General practitioners may delegate care to CAM practitioners employed by the practice, or to another therapist, but must be sure that the treatment is appropriate for the patient and likely to be of benefit. The general practitioner needs to continue to monitor the patient's progress and ensure the patient has access to any conventional treatment that is required (BMA 1999, Zollman & Vickers 1999a).

Teamworking

How can we make shared care work?

Doctors referring patients for CAM or delegating care will transfer appropriate clinical information to the therapist (with the patient's consent). Therapists should endeavour to liaise effectively with the patient's general practitioner, and with other colleagues if working in the context of a multidisciplinary team. Patients referring themselves for complementary therapy should be encouraged to inform their general practitioner and to continue to attend there for review. Good patient records should be made and retained by all CAM therapists. The therapist should not alter a patient's medication or treatment without prior consultation and agreement from the patient's doctor. Any adverse reactions to treatment should be reported and recorded in the patient's medical record (Zollman & Vickers 1999a, Frenkel & Borkan 2003).

If a patient remains insistent on seeing a complementary therapist rather than following advice that conventional treatment is needed, the doctor should record this information clearly in the patient's record (BMA 1999).

Despite significant barriers, including attitudes and beliefs among conventional practitioners and concerns about the lack of scientific evidence for some CAM, many therapists have expressed a wish to be viewed as offering complementary rather than alternative care. They would like to work more closely with doctors and other healthcare professionals in seeking to deliver holistic, accessible, patient-centred and integrated healthcare (Barrett et al 2004). Integration will, however, depend on both conventional and CAM practitioners being educated in a way that enables them to communicate and to understand not just the clinical practice of the other discipline but the language and concepts used to describe it (Caspi et al 2000) (Fig. 29). Conventional practitioners need to increase their ability to evaluate, describe and explain CAM, and complementary practitioners would do well to consider the benefits of robust assessment of efficacy and audit of outcomes.

Summary

It is possible and desirable for CAM to be better integrated into conventional medical care. For this to occur, doctors

Key points

- Doctors should always ask patients about CAM use as part of history taking.
- Most patients want their doctor to initiate a discussion about CAM and welcome information and advice.
- Doctors need to have adequate knowledge about CAM and local CAM therapists to be able to discuss it fully as part of shared decision-making and treatment planning.
- Doctors and reputable CAM therapists will seek to work together and communicate effectively so that patients gain maximum benefit from CAM and conventional medicine.

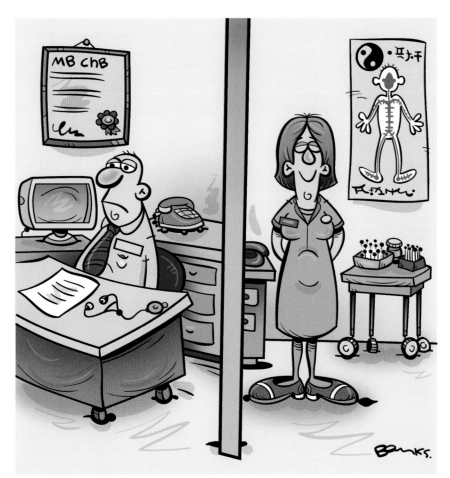

Fig. 29 **'I find it so difficult to communicate with other practitioners.'**

need to be better informed about the therapies available in their locality, able to provide information, advice and support to patients considering or already using CAM, and aware of their ethical and legal obligations.

Therapists need to be registered where possible, to follow a code of practice that includes accurate assessment, regular review of planned care, and effective collaboration and liaison with the patient's doctor.

Specific CAM therapies

Manual medicine

James P. M. Campbell

What is manual medicine?

Manual medicine is a form of physical therapy involving the use of the therapist's hands (generally) on the body of a patient to produce structural change that induces a healing benefit. It is practised by various professional groups, including some doctors and most physiotherapists, but it is the principal treatment modality employed by chiropractic and osteopathy.

Chiropractic and osteopathy are both manipulation-based therapies. The two therapies have much in common but chiropractors tend to focus on the joints of the spine and nervous system while osteopaths put equal emphasis on the joints and surrounding muscles, tendons and ligaments.

The underlying belief is that many health problems are caused by faulty mechanical function of the body and this faulty function can be corrected by physical treatment. Misalignment of spinal joints may be caused by a past injury or postural stress.

Osteopaths and chiropractors mainly treat back and neck pain but also treat a range of other problems including digestive disorders, asthma and sports injuries.

History

Manipulation (manual therapy) has a long history. It was used in ancient Greece, and 'bonesetters' were part of all early Eastern and European traditions. Hippocrates refers to manipulation as an old art.

However, there was little formal development of physical treatments (compared with pharmacology and surgery) until the creation of osteopathy and chiropractic, which both have their origins in late 19th century Midwestern America.

A. T. Still was a physician who developed a new treatment paradigm based on the musculoskeletal system as a key to the diagnosis and treatment of disease.

D. D. Palmer was a self-educated healer who founded chiropractic in Davenport, Iowa, believing that spinal dysfunction was the basis of most disease and that correction of the dysfunction could cure all.

High- and low-velocity thrust techniques, gentle rotations, mobilisations and stretches are all used in order to release muscle tension, reduce joint stiffness and improve circulation.

Many doctors have developed an interest in manipulation, particularly in Europe. Mennell in the 1950s was an important pioneer and protagonist of osteopathic techniques. His disciple, Cyriax, wrote the *Textbook of Orthopaedic Medicine* in 1978. Stoddart was a medical graduate and also a Doctor of Osteopathy (DO) and wrote the *Manual of Osteopathic Technique* in 1961. The London College of Osteopathic Medicine (LCOM) was the first institute where osteopathic techniques were taught to qualified doctors. Hundreds of doctors in Germany, Switzerland, Austria, Holland and Scandinavia have learnt manual techniques through training courses. Developments in Eastern Europe have been less hampered by professional divisions, according to Lewit (1991). In the United Kingdom the professional organisation for doctors practising manipulation is the British Institute of Musculoskeletal Medicine (BIMM).

Underlying philosophy

Both osteopathy and chiropractic share a common philosophy:

- the body functions as a unit
- structure and function are interrelated
- the body has an inherent ability to heal itself
- when normal adaptability is disrupted disease can ensue.

Chiropractors generally use rapid forceful movements, termed high-velocity thrusts, designed to realign and mobilise the spine. This form of manipulation may produce a clicking sound.

Osteopaths also carry out high-velocity thrusts but in addition use a range of other techniques including stretching, massage, mobilisation and release techniques (called muscle energy technique – MET).

What is the difference between osteopathy and chiropractic?

Osteopathy and chiropractic have different historical origins and have evolved along separate paths, although with significant overlap with regard to philosophy and practice. Osteopathy is not limited to thrust techniques. Soft tissue and visceral techniques are common. Chiropractic focuses primarily on thrust techniques applied to the spine. Chiropractors traditionally use X-rays as part of their assessment, not only to identify pathology but also to measure structural alignment.

The role of manipulation within conventional medicine

The UK BEAM trial (2004a, 2004b) compared the effect of adding manipulation and/or exercise classes to best GP care for patients presenting with low back pain. Manipulation was found to improve outcomes in both the short and longer term. The economic analysis indicated that manipulation was a cost-effective addition to 'best care' in general practice. The manipulation treatment in this study was provided by osteopaths, chiropractors and physiotherapists.

Evidence of efficacy and safety

The most serious potential risks of osteopathic or chiropractic treatments are spinal cord injury or stroke after neck manipulation. This is a rare complication, with estimates varying from one in 70 000 treatments to one in 5 million.

Less severe but more common side effects include discomfort and pain. Forceful manipulation should be avoided in subjects with osteoporosis and (traditionally) during pregnancy.

Pros and cons of manipulation

The use of manipulative therapy for some purposes enjoys wide acceptance by medical authorities in many nations, and is covered by many health insurance plans. However, it is not widely available in the UK National Health Service. The incorporation of physiotherapists into the NHS but not other physical therapy professions has happened more by chance than design.

The emphasis on disturbed mechanical function rather than pathology may be at odds with the traditional 'disease model' of medicine but is more in keeping with more holistic and mind–body models.

Many patients seen in hospital outpatient clinics with unexplained symptoms are probably exhibiting 'disordered function' and this is frequently the case with musculoskeletal pains.

Diagnosis of spinal dysfunction

When examining a patient with a mechanical pain problem the diagnosis often relies on physical examination and palpation of the affected tissues. The manual therapist will diagnose dysfunction of the spine by looking for Asymmetry, Range of movement abnormality and Tissue tension abnormality (ART).

Principles of manipulation

The active range of joint movement is depicted in Figure 30 as an arc either side of a neutral position. When an examiner checks the passive range of joint movement this will usually be found to be greater than the active range. Treatments involving passive joint movement within this physiological range are termed 'mobilisation'. If a joint is forcefully taken beyond this physiological range (into the paraphysiological zone) then 'manipulation' occurs (Fig. 30). Forceful attempts to take the joint beyond this zone will

result in ligament strains and other potential tissue damage. High-velocity thrust (HVT) techniques must also include low amplitude (LA) to avoid this.

Figure 31 shows the effect of placing increasing longitudinal tension on a finger (interphalangeal) joint. At a certain level of tension the joint surfaces suddenly separate and an audible 'crack' is produced with release of nitrogen gas in the joint. Following the 'crack' there is an increase in passive range of joint movement but the gas bubble is slowly absorbed and the 'load–separation' curve loops back to the starting position.

Sources of further information

- British Institute of Musculoskeletal Medicine: www.bimm.org.uk
- Greenman P 2003 Principles of manual medicine, 3rd edn. Williams & Wilkins, Baltimore
- Lewit K 1999 Manipulative therapy in rehabilitation of the locomotor system, 3rd edn. Butterworth Heinemann, Oxford
- London College of Osteopathic Medicine: 8–10 Boston Place, London NW1 6QH

 STOP THINK
- In what ways are osteopathy, chiropractic and manual medicine 'complementary' or 'alternative'?
- Lay practitioners may work to different philosophies from mainstream medicine (e.g. chiropractic reliance on X-rays for positional diagnosis).
- Should any form of treatment with evidence-based benefit be used (appropriately) by the medical profession?

Key points

- Chiropractic and osteopathy are both manipulation-based therapies.
- Manipulation is also used by some doctors and physiotherapists.
- Bodily structure and function are interrelated and disordered function can be treated by manipulative techniques.
- Manipulation is only one type of physical medicine treatment.

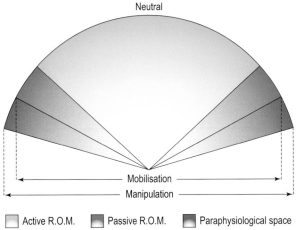

Fig. 30 **Joint manipulation and mobilisation.** ROM, range of movement.

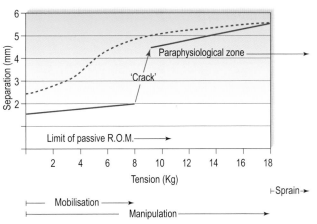

Fig. 31 **Load separation curve.**

Osteopathy

James P. M. Campbell

What is osteopathy?

Osteopathy is a system of detecting and treating parts of the body that are malfunctioning or damaged. It primarily uses manual therapy and relies on palpation to detect altered function.

It utilises the concept that the body is a self-regulating mechanism, that structure and function are interrelated, and that altered function can be corrected by restoring structural integrity.

What is osteopathy used for?

Patients seek osteopathic treatment predominantly for musculoskeletal pain problems, such as back and neck pain, sports injuries and headaches. Some practitioners offer mechanical treatments or cranial treatments for any type of disorder including infant colic, asthma and irritable bowel syndrome. In a government report on back pain (Clinical Standards Advisory Group 1994) it was estimated that osteopaths spent 67% of their time on low back pain treatment.

History

Osteopathy was founded in America in 1874 by Dr Andrew Taylor Still in Kirksville, Missouri (Fig. 32). He was the son of a doctor and went to medical school for formal training. During his early years of medical practice he noticed how his patients' health was influenced by the way they used their bodies. He devised a new method of physical treatment to address this. Teaching of osteopathy began in 1892 and practitioners arrived in the UK at the start of the 20th century to practise osteopathy and set up a school of osteopathy in London in 1917. There were tensions between osteopathy and the medical profession in Britain for many years, and 25 years ago it was considered a disciplinary offence for a general practitioner to recommend osteopathic treatment to patients. This situation has steadily improved and, particularly since its statutory regulation, osteopathy is recognised as one of the three main disciplines of physical therapy.

The scope of osteopathic treatment

Osteopaths will assess their patients by history and examination. Movement tests (e.g. spinal segmental motion testing) and palpation of tissues are the primary assessment methods with little use of investigations, such as X-rays. Developing skill with palpation requires repeated exposure to both normal and abnormal findings. As medical investigations become more sophisticated, basic examination skills tend to assume less importance, but with problems of disturbed mechanical function (very common cause of musculoskeletal symptoms) investigations will generally be normal and only careful clinical examination will allow proper diagnosis. The process of examination itself is often therapeutic – therapeutic touch!

A visit to the osteopath

Following a full case history, examination will involve a series of movement tests and palpation of tissues. Differences from standard orthopaedic examination will include assessment of movement at individual segments in the spine and examination of muscle trigger points. Treatments involve soft tissue techniques, joint mobilisations, release techniques and high-velocity thrust techniques (Fig. 33).

Present regulation

Osteopathy and chiropractic are currently the only CAM therapies covered by statutory regulation. The title 'osteopath'

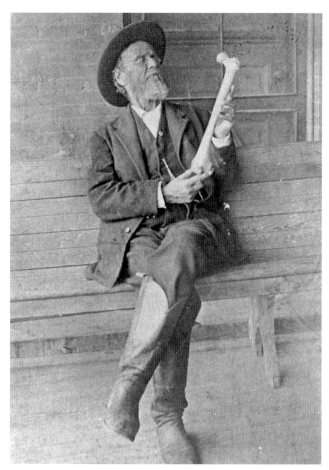

Fig. 32 **Dr A. T. Still – founder of osteopathy.** (Reproduced courtesy of Still National Osteopathic Museum and National Center for Osteopathy, Kirksville, MO.)

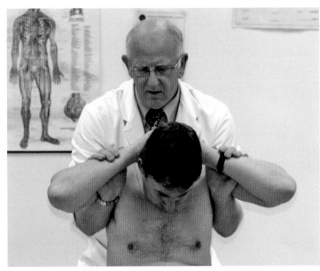

Fig. 33 **Osteopathic practitioner.** (Courtesy of General Osteopathic Council, Kampfner copyright.)

became protected by law in May 2000. It is now a criminal offence to describe oneself as an osteopath in the UK unless registered with the General Osteopathic Council (see Section 2).

In order to join the Register of Osteopaths practitioners have to complete a course of approved training, such as a 4-year degree level course, and satisfy the General Osteopathic Council they have reached the required standards of safety and competency. Registered osteopaths also have to maintain professional indemnity insurance cover.

Role within conventional medicine

In the US osteopathy, through its educational process and licensing, has become virtually indistinguishable from allopathic medicine. Doctors of Osteopathy (DOs) have full medical practice rights along with MDs (conventionally trained doctors) and many seldom utilise the manipulative origins of their background. However, in the UK osteopathy firmly remains a physical therapy profession.

The majority of osteopaths work as independent practitioners and are consulted privately by people with various problems, most commonly spinal pain.

Their training and experience allow osteopaths to identify when possible serious pathology might be present and when to refer the patient to their general practitioner for further investigation.

Range of treatments

Stretching of tight muscles and exercises for weak muscles can be used along with soft tissue massage-type treatments and joint mobilisations. Efficient stretching can be achieved with muscle energy technique (MET) where active contraction of the muscle group to be stretched is followed by its passive stretching in a cycle. High-velocity, low-amplitude thrusts may be used. Mobilisations may involve 'accessory movements' where joints are moved in non-physiological directions.

Although spinal treatments comprise the bulk of general osteopathic practice, dysfunction of peripheral joints can often be helped by mobilising treatment.

What is the evidence for osteopathic treatment?

Clinical trials have shown minimal to moderate evidence of short-term relief in low back pain. Some benefit has been shown for migraine, tension headache and neck pain but no effect has been demonstrated in asthma, hypertension or dysmenorrhoea. There have been no studies comparing different manipulative techniques.

Why do people in the UK pay to visit osteopaths?

Osteopaths and chiropractors provide a form of therapy that is not generally available to NHS patients. Accordingly people with acute and chronic musculoskeletal disorders will frequently be prepared to see a private practitioner for help with their problem. Most physiotherapists do not offer the same type of treatment. However, osteopaths, chiropractors and other private practitioners are generally seeing the subgroup of individuals who are interested and motivated to get better, whereas NHS practice tends also to include those with different agendas (e.g. secondary gain, presentation of psychosocial distress with physical symptoms, employment and medicolegal issues).

Sources of further information

- General Osteopathic Council: www.osteopathy.org.uk
- UK BEAM Trial Team 2004 United Kingdom back pain exercise and manipulation (UK BEAM) randomised trial: cost effectiveness of physical treatments for back pain in primary care. BMJ 329:1381. (Manipulation is cost-effective)
- UK BEAM Trial Team 2004 United Kingdom back pain exercise and manipulation (UK BEAM) randomised trial: effectiveness of physical treatments for back pain in primary care. BMJ 329:1377. (Small/moderate but significant benefits from manipulation and exercise compared with other 'best care')

 STOP THINK

- Cranial osteopathy (or craniosacral therapy) is a controversial subcategory of osteopathy that uses a very gentle adjustment of cranial bones or therapeutic touch to influence the ebb and flow of the CSF. The scientific basis and efficacy of cranial osteopathy remains to be established.

Key points

- Osteopathy is primarily a system of detecting and treating symptoms arising from mechanical malfunction.
- Only practitioners on the UK Register of Osteopaths may call themselves an osteopath.

Chiropractic

James P. M. Campbell

What is chiropractic?

Chiropractic is concerned with the diagnosis, treatment and prevention of mechanical disorders of the musculoskeletal system and the effects of these disorders on the function of the nervous system and general health. There is an emphasis on manual treatments including spinal manipulation or 'adjustment' (World Federation of Chiropractic 1999). The word 'chiropractic' is derived from the Greek words *cheira* (hand) and *praxis* (action).

Chiropractic focuses on the spine as integral to maintaining health through maintenance of optimal neurophysiological balance. Faulty spinal function (often termed 'subluxations') can be addressed through chiropractic 'adjustment'.

Chiropractic is most often used to treat musculoskeletal conditions – problems with the muscles, joints, bones, and connective tissues such as cartilage, ligaments and tendons. In the US 3–16% of adults receive chiropractic manipulation each year.

History of chiropractic

Chiropractic was developed in 1895, in Davenport, Iowa, by Daniel D. Palmer (Fig. 34). He was a self-educated healer who believed that spinal dysfunction was the basis of most disease and that correction of the dysfunction could cure all.

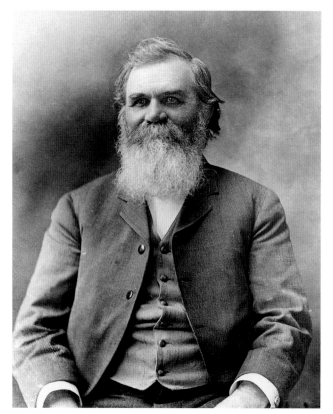

Fig. 34 **D. D. Palmer – founder of chiropractic.** (Reproduced courtesy of Palmer College of Chiropractic Archives.)

He famously restored someone's hearing by noticing a swelling in the spine and reducing this malalignment by manipulation.

Chiropractic has developed over the last century with spread of its practitioners to many parts of the world.

Present regulation

The Chiropractors Act 1994 established the General Chiropractic Council (GCC) to regulate the profession. Since June 2001 'chiropractor' has been a protected title and it is a criminal offence to describe oneself as a chiropractor unless registered with the GCC.

The title 'doctor' is unprotected but generally understood by the general public to indicate a medical practitioner or someone with a higher 'doctorate' degree. Many chiropractors award themselves this courtesy title! Generally chiropractors will have undertaken a BSc degree course, or equivalent.

What is chiropractic used for?

Low back pain, neck pain and headache are common indications for chiropractic treatment. The GCC patient leaflet also indicates that conditions such as asthma, digestive disorders, migraine, infant colic and menstrual pain can be treated. Some practitioners believe that most disease can relate to spinal disorder and is therefore treatable by chiropractic adjustment.

In a government report on back pain (Clinical Standards Advisory Group 1994) it was estimated that chiropractors spent 50% of their time treating low back pain.

Classical chiropractic theory denies otherwise accepted medical facts about the origin of diseases, and instead holds that the correction of subluxation can cure or treat most disease. Although manipulative therapy has been shown to have some efficacy in treating back pain, headache, and other symptoms of spinal-related conditions, few rigorous studies have supported the efficacy of chiropractic medicine outside of this specific area.

How do chiropractors assess their patients?

At an initial visit to a chiropractor you would undergo a history and examination with particular emphasis on the spine. Palpation is used to find spinal segments that are 'subluxed' and hence not functioning normally.

You may also undergo X-ray examination. A treatment plan is then developed. Treatment involves 'adjustments' or manipulation treatment. A controlled sudden force is applied, usually to the spine. For an acute problem three treatments a week may be advised, with longer intervals between further treatments depending on the nature of the problem and the patient's response.

Chiropractic places a lot of emphasis on radiological assessment. This remains at odds with current medical opinion and its appreciation of the limited value of X-rays in conditions such as low back pain, and the poor correlation between X-ray findings and symptoms. Spinal X-rays often involve quite large doses of radiation and therefore their use needs to be justified.

Treatment philosophy

Chiropractic philosophy believes that correction of faulty spinal function followed by maintenance of good function is central to good health. This is achieved by manipulative therapy (Fig. 35). The 'find it, fix it, and leave it alone' approach of most osteopathic practice is in contrast to the chiropractic approach of ongoing maintenance treatment to prevent problems.

The role of chiropractic within conventional medicine

Chiropractic has always maintained its independence from 'mainstream medicine'. Many practitioners offer chiropractic treatment for a wide range of complaints beyond those associated with disordered mechanical function.

Evidence of efficacy and safety

The mechanisms underlying chiropractic manipulation have been studied in animal models and the forces involved have been measured in cadavers and normal volunteers (Pickar 2002, Swenson & Haldeman 2003).

Risks have to be evaluated relative to the seriousness of the condition and likely benefit. Manipulation of the neck can have serious consequences (vertebral artery damage leading to stroke and paralysis) and lumbar manipulations may lead to aggravation of an acute disc prolapse.

Some chiropractors believe that every spine will benefit potentially from manipulation (or adjustment) and hence the need for long-term maintenance treatment. Although treatment risks may be small, in the absence of symptoms the risk/benefit balance suggests this belief may not be justified.

Clinical trials of manipulative therapies pose certain difficulties. How do you identify a reproducible intervention and its 'dose' and frequency? What is an appropriate control group (what is sham manipulation?)? There is a problem blinding the subjects and the therapists, and a problem with valid outcome measures.

The trial by Meade and colleagues (1995) comparing chiropractic treatment for low back pain and standard NHS physiotherapy treatment is often quoted in support of the superiority of chiropractic treatment. However, there were many confounding factors (e.g. the physiotherapists tended to be relatively junior and the chiropractors saw patients in more pleasant surroundings in their private clinics).

A general review of the scientific evidence for the effectiveness of chiropractic manipulation for back pain by Ernst (2003) concluded that results 'have not tended to be encouraging' and the evidence is 'at best uncertain'.

Sources of further information

■ British Chiropractic Association: www.chiropractic-uk.co.uk
■ General Chiropractic Council (UK): www.gcc-uk.org
■ Some sceptical views on chiropractic: www.//chirobase.org

Case study

Active versus passive treatment

Some physical treatments (e.g. heat) are mainly palliative whereas exercise therapy can bring about positive change in mechanical function. Manual therapy is a passive treatment and may work best when combined with exercise and lifestyle change. Especially with chronic or recurrent conditions the patient should ideally be involved as an active participant in treatment.

■ Can current orthodox medical advice to limit ionising radiation be compatible with the traditional use of X-rays in chiropractic to diagnose structural changes?
■ Is structural asymmetry always abnormal?
■ What is the difference between *active* treatments and *passive* treatments?

Key points

■ Chiropractic diagnosis and treatment is concerned primarily with spinal function and its effects on the nervous system.
■ Treatment usually involves spinal manipulation (high-velocity thrust techniques).
■ The profession is regulated in the UK by Act of Parliament.

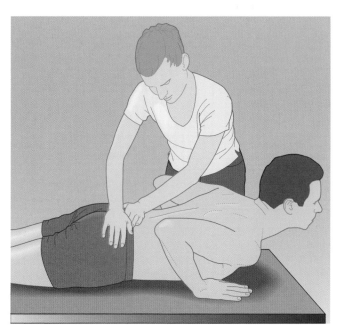

Fig. 35 **Manipulation.**

Herbal medicine

David Brown

What is it?

A system of medicine which uses various remedies derived from plants and plant extracts to treat disorders and maintain good health. Another term for this type of treatment is phytotherapy.

Background

Plant material has been used to treat illness for thousands of years. Initially, primitive man would self-treat on a trial and error basis but later medical care became organised with local healers and the sharing of information. The first written record of the use of herbs was in 2800 BC in China, the Pen Ts'ao. It is claimed that Chinese herbalism derived from the Ayurveda system in India. In Europe, the Greeks then the Romans wrote herbal texts. From 800 AD, monks in northern Europe were cultivating and using medicinal herbs. The primacy of herbal medicine was only challenged in the early 19th century by mineral-based treatments such as mercurials. The modern pharmaceutical industry, from the beginning of the 20th century, made possible by the development of industrial-scale chemical technology, was based on the analysis of the active ingredients of plants and the modification of these molecules for increased efficacy and safety. Twenty-five per cent of modern medicines are derived from plants.

Do we need herbal medicines?

In the Western World, the use of herbal medicines remains widespread. Over 30% of the British population use herbal medicine, spending in excess of £50 million annually (Ernst & White 2000). In Germany, 70% of physicians prescribe herbal medicines and in Europe in 1991, over-the-counter sales of herbal products amounted to £1.41 billion. Global spending on herbal medicines is $60 billion (WHO 2003) (Table 16).

The WHO (2003) estimate that 80% of the world's population still rely on traditional medicine for some aspects of their primary care (Fig. 36). Patients in the developing world lack the wealth to access modern pharmaceuticals. It is a priority in these countries to develop affordable sources of effective therapies and, to this end, the WHO is sponsoring studies to assess herbal remedies such as artemisia in the treatment of malaria. It is also important to ensure the sustainable cultivation of these plants.

There is continued exploration of Third World herbal remedies for agents that might have commercial use in the Western world. *Hoodia gordonii* (Fig. 37), a succulent growing wild in the Kalahari Desert, has been used for centuries by the Bushmen as an appetite suppressant. *Hoodia* extract is now being marketed here as an aid to dieting.

Regulation and training

In the UK, relatively few medical practitioners practise herbal medicine. Herbal remedies are purchased from pharmacists, by mail order or, with or without a consultation, from a herbalist. As yet, there is no regulatory body for or compulsory registration of herbalists. The National Institute of Medical Herbalists has been in existence since 1864 and provides voluntary registration for those who have undergone a 3-year training course. As this registration is not statutory, anyone, with or without training or experience, can legitimately

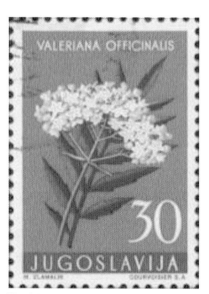
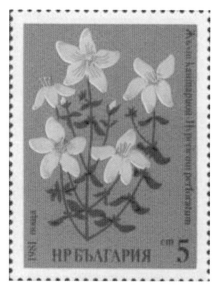
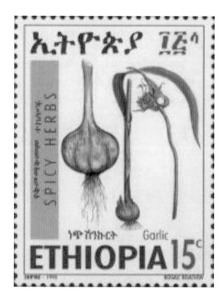

Fig. 36 **Philatelic collection of herbal plants from various countries.**

Table 16	**Top selling herbal medications in the UK**
Usually sole agents	Echinacea
	Panax ginseng
	Ginkgo biloba
	St John's wort
Usually in combinations with other herbs	Valerian
	Garlic
	Passiflora
	Senna

set up business as a herbalist. Legislation is currently being proposed and formulated to amend this situation. University courses now exist to provide graduate courses in medical herbalism, with teaching in anatomy, physiology and pharmacology.

Herbal products are used mainly for minor illnesses such as upper respiratory infections and for rheumatic, menopausal or sleep problems (Table 17).

Issues surrounding use of herbal medicines

There is no doubt that extracts of foxglove (digitalis) or deadly nightshade (atropine) have considerable and potentially fatal effects. Other traditional remedies have a use that can be rationalised by modern chemical analysis. Chasteberry (*Vitex agnus castus*) was used, among other purposes, to suppress the libido of medieval monks and has been shown to contain phytoestrogens. This herb and others have a rationale for their medicinal use.

There are problems in conducting clinical research into herbal products for two main reasons.

1. Herbalists tend not to prescribe single remedies but rather provide mixtures of five or six herbal extracts, often varying the proportions of the mixture at each consultation to reflect the change in symptoms. They also knowingly

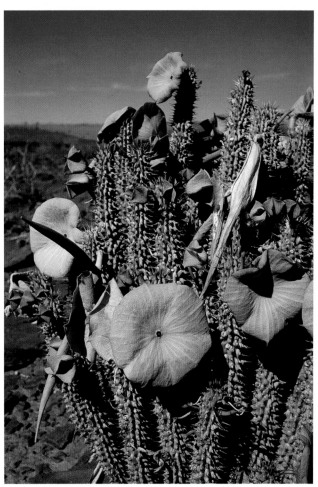

Fig. 37 ***Hoodia gordonii* plant.** (Photograph courtesy of Colin Paterson, Natural Visions.)

prescribe in what conventional pharmacology would consider subtherapeutic doses, as their aim is symptom reduction, thereby enabling the body to heal itself.

Table 17	**Examples of benefits as shown by clinical trials**		
Herb	**Indication**	**Benefit**	**Comment**
Chasteberry (*Vitex agnus castus*)	Premenstrual tension	All symptoms except bloating	One trial only. 3 month double-blind clinical and self-assessment
Echinacea	Urinary tract infections	Slight reduction in duration and severity of cold	Only when taken immediately at onset of symptoms. No preventive benefit
Evening primrose	Mastalgia	Small benefit over placebo	No trials show benefit in premenstrual syndrome or in symptoms of menopause
	Rheumatoid arthritis	Improved signs and symptoms of disease	High dosage over more than 6 months usage
Feverfew	Prevention of migraine	Reduced frequency of headache compared to placebo in classical migraine	Benefit after a few weeks treatment; use fresh or dried leaves not alcoholic extract. Rebound of headaches on discontinuation
Garlic	Hypercholesterolaemia	Improved lipid profile versus placebo not sustained beyond 6 months	No significant effect on blood pressure
Ginger	Nausea, vomiting	Nausea not of central origin, e.g. gastrointestinal irritation	?Role in morning sickness
Ginkgo	Claudication	Significant dose-related benefit versus placebo after 24 weeks	Benefit about 35 metres improvement in claudication distance
	Dementia	Significant slight benefit versus placebo. 6 month delay in progression	Slightly better in Alzheimer's than in vascular dementia
Horse chestnut seed	Chronic venous insufficiency	Significant improvement in leg volume versus placebo	Comparable benefit to grade 2 stockings
Saw palmetto	Symptoms of benign prostatic hypertrophy	Similar benefit in trials versus finasteride	Fewer side effects, e.g. impotence. Ensure malignancy excluded before use
St John's wort	Mild to moderate depression	Similar benefit to low-dose tricyclics. Fewer side effects	Less effective than SSRIs in moderate to severe depression. Interactions, adverse effects
Valerian	Insomnia	Mild hypnotic. Similar to benzodiazepines	Headache and grogginess in morning. Possible acute withdrawal symptoms

2. It is difficult to manufacture a consistent standardised herbal product. The timing of harvesting, when the herb is ripe and even the correct time of day will affect the quality of the herbal extract. Obtaining the herb from a reliable producer is important to ensure that the correct herb is used. Problems can occur with wild collected plants, especially in the developing world. Substitution can be either deliberate or accidental and contamination with animal material or heavy metals can also occur. Testing for bioequivalence can be done by assay for a particular component by mass spectrometry. This may not be a true indicator of equivalence as that marker may not be the only or main active ingredient. Hypericin is the marker for St John's wort (Fig. 38) but it is known that hyperforin is also a potent constituent. It has been shown that the proportions of these two components are not constant and can be affected by the ripeness of the plant at harvesting. Extracts may also have the marker ingredient added to comply with the assay but may be deficient in other active components.

These factors make rigorous controlled studies near impossible. In addition, herbalists argue that such trials would not truly reflect the holistic, interactive one-to-one basis of herbal practice. 'Big business' herbal producers who predominantly manufacture monotherapies say they cannot afford to conduct clinical trials.

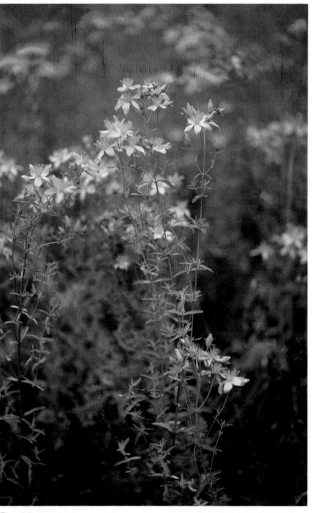

Fig. 38 **St John's wort.** (Photograph courtesy of Heather Angel, Natural Visions.)

What evidence exists?

Evidence is available at several levels of statistical significance. The most available and most numerous source is unscientific 'folklore', the anecdotal, experience-based information which is found in magazine articles, websites and the popular media. This information is used mainly to promote sales of herbal products and encourages their perception as natural and safe. Concern has also been expressed that some sources of information not only advocate an alternative remedy but discourage patients with serious conditions from taking their conventional treatments.

Many of the randomised controlled trials (RCTs) into herbal monotherapies have been sponsored by the large herbal manufacturers. It is debatable whether this may introduce an element of bias into the reporting of the results; trials that show a poor or negative outcome may not be submitted for publication. An analysis of trials published in journals of alternative medicine in 1995 showed that only 1% produced negative results. Little has changed, in that a similar review in 2000 showed this had increased only to 5% negative results (Schmidt et al 2001).

There have been relatively few rigorously controlled studies into the efficacy of herbal products. For example, trials have shown a significant benefit in symptoms of dementia when treated with *Ginkgo biloba* extract. This was based on assessment by carers. The benefit, however, was not observed in another study where the characteristic bitter taste of *Ginkgo biloba* was controlled for by using quinine as the placebo (Ernst & Pittler 1999).

The choice is whether to investigate one aspect of treatment in a simple, conventional trial or to make the effort to design a trial that will reflect the reality of the whole therapeutic process. In the US the National Center for Complementary and Alternative Medicine (NCCAM) was set up in 2000 to 'explore complementary and alternative healing practices in the context of rigorous science, to educate and train CAM researchers and to disseminate authoritative information to the public and professionals'. It was given a budget of $68 million for the first year. It is accepted that it must prioritise its efforts and, in the herbal field, it has supported ongoing trials into St John's wort for depression, *Ginkgo biloba* in Alzheimer's disease and saw palmetto for benign prostatic hypertrophy, areas where some evidence of efficacy along with adverse effects and interactions have been noted. These trials are designed to overcome the deficiencies, identified by meta-analyses of previous studies in these areas, of size and duration of studies. The above studies will be traditional RCTs but others will be conducted comparing different treatment systems in their entirety, with clear clinical end points. This is appropriate for holistic treatment systems where the 'active ingredient' is undefined.

Evidence of efficacy

Relatively few herbal products have been shown to have significant benefit in properly conducted randomised control trials. However, St John's wort has been shown to be as effective as low-dose tricyclic antidepressants and has fewer side effects in the treatment of mild to moderate depression (Linde et al 1996). In Ireland St John's wort is classified as a medicinal product and therefore, only available on prescription. For severe depression, a NCCAM study (Hypericum Depression

Trial Study Group 2002) has shown that it is no better at relieving symptoms than placebo.

Saw palmetto has been shown to have similar benefits to finasteride in treating benign prostatic hypertrophy and again has fewer side effects (Wilt et al 1999). *Ginkgo biloba* may have a slight benefit in improving walking distance in claudication (Pittler & Ernst 2000). Garlic produces an improved lipid profile compared to placebo but the benefit is not sustained beyond 6 months (Stevinson et al 2000).

Studies of other popular herbal remedies have failed to show any benefit. These include evening primrose for mastalgia and premenstrual symptoms (Chenoy et al 1994), garlic for blood pressure and ginseng (Fig. 39) for any condition. Echinacea is a widely used herb, particularly for the prevention of upper respiratory infections. Some trials have shown a marginal reduction in the duration of symptoms of coryza when echinacea is started immediately at onset (Melchart et al 1999). However, a recent study by the NCCAM on echinacea in children showed no benefit when used in this way (NCCAM 2004).

Safety issues

Treatment of an illness usually follows on from a process of consultation with a professional, investigations and a discussion of the risks and benefits of intervention. Self-treatment removes several of the safeguards built into this process. For example, self-medicating with over-the-counter saw palmetto may expose a man with prostatic symptoms to the risk of not having a malignancy detected. This risk can be diminished by consulting a herbalist who acknowledges the potential hazards of treatment without diagnosis and who feels able to communicate with the patient's doctor.

Side effects

- Most herbal products probably have minimal side effects, comparable to placebo in trials.
- Garlic can cause odour.
- St John's wort can cause photosensitisation, particularly in the fair-skinned.
- Feverfew, used to treat migraine, can cause, on discontinuation, a rebound of headache plus anxiety and insomnia.

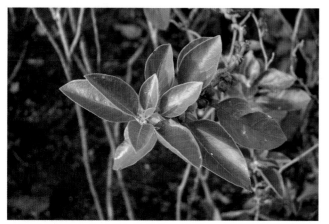

Fig. 39 **Ginseng.**

- Valerian, a popular herbal hypnotic, can result in morning grogginess and headache.

More serious side effects:

- Case reports of subdural (Rowin & Lewis 1996) and subarachnoid haemorrhage (Vale 1998) associated with the use of *Ginkgo biloba*.
- Kava-kava, a herbal anxiolytic, is the subject of a voluntary ban in the UK because of reported hepatotoxicity (Brauer et al 2003).

Poorer quality products may, ironically, cause fewer problems if they contain less active ingredient.

Safety also relates to the quality of the manufacturing process. Does the product contain the claimed ingredients? Analysis of samples in the US showed that only 25% actually contained the purported ingredient, ginseng (Liberti & Der Marderosian 1978) (see issue of adulteration in Chinese herbal medicine section).

Interaction of herbal products with conventional medications is a major issue. Since 1996, the Medicines and Healthcare products Regulation Agency (MHRA) in the UK has collected data on herb/drug interactions via the Yellow Card reporting scheme. It is likely that there is considerable under-reporting. Even with conventional medicines, the MHRA estimate that only 10–15% of serious adverse drug reactions (ADRs) are reported. It is likely that this figure is even lower with herbals. In the UK, Barnes and colleagues (1998) found that patients would be much less liable to consult their GP about an ADR to a herbal product than to a conventional medicine. Ninety per cent of patients questioned believed that it was safe to mix herbal and conventional medicines.

The majority of patients (72%) will not disclose to their physician that they are taking a herbal product, either because they are not taking it for the condition they are consulting with or because of concern that the physician might disapprove (Kaye et al 2000).

St John's wort is believed to induce hepatic cytochrome P450 and is thereby capable of reducing the efficacy of the combined oral contraceptive pill (COCP), theophylline, ciclosporin, anticonvulsants such as carbamazepine, phenobarbital and phenytoin, triptans and protease inhibitors. The effect of St John's wort on digoxin is by a different route, by the induction of the p-glycoprotein drug transporter, causing a decrease in digoxin levels. Data from the Committee on Safety of Medicines (CSM) show that the most common interactions reported have been between St John's wort and COCPs, causing both intermenstrual bleeding and unplanned pregnancies. The data sheets enclosed with warfarin and COCPs contain warnings about concomitant use of St John's wort.

Other possible interactions are listed in Table 18.

Summary

Herbal remedies have been used worldwide since the beginning of history. Many of these products have been subsumed into conventional medicine. They are obtainable over-the-counter or through a herbalist. Their use continues as an alternative to conventional medicine. In the developing world, economics determine their primacy and require their exploration for cheap alternatives to costly pharmaceuticals. In the developed world, they appeal to consumers as an alternative to the high-tech healthcare system and continue to represent a potential source of novel pharmaceuticals. Compared to synthetic drugs, herbal medicines exhibit low potency and a relatively low incidence of adverse effects. There is little quality evidence for their efficacy. They are, however, not impotent and can cause adverse effects and interact with conventional medicine.

Sources of further information

- Barnes J, Anderson L, Phillipson D 2002 Herbal medicines: a guide for healthcare professionals, 2nd edn. Pharmaceutical Press, London. (Very good reference book on various herbal medicines)
- Edwards I R, Aronson J K 2000 Adverse drug reactions: definitions, diagnosis and management. Lancet 356(9237):1255–1259

- Licensing of medicines: policy on herbal medicine. Online. Available: www.mhra.gov.uk/home, under 'How we regulate' June 2005
- Medicines and Healthcare products Regulatory Agency: http://medicines.mhra.gov.uk. (The agency responsible for the administration and enforcement of medicine legislation in the UK)

STOP THINK
- Are the active ingredients in herbal medicines present in sufficient quantity and consistency to be considered therapeutic?
- A conventional medicine is subjected to rigorous and expensive RCTs and clinical trials before approval. What is the evidence for a herbal product?

Table 18 **Examples of possible herb–drug interactions**

Drug	Herbal product	Interaction
Alcohol	Valerian, kava-kava	Increased sedation
Anticonvulsants:		
Barbiturates	Valerian, kava-kava	Increased sedation
	St John's wort	Loss of seizure control
Phenytoin	Evening primrose, St John's wort	Loss of seizure control
Antidepressants:		
Selective serotonin reuptake inhibitors (SSRIs)	St John's wort	Serotonin syndrome (agitation, tremor, palpitations and gastrointestinal upset)
MAOIs	*Panax ginseng*	Headache, tremor, manic
Aspirin	Feverfew, garlic, ginkgo, ginger	Decreased platelet aggregation, prolonged bleeding time
Benzodiazepines	Valerian, kava-kava	Increased sedation
	St John's wort	Reduced ciclosporin blood levels and transplant rejection
	Echinacea	Theoretical risk of reduction in immunosuppressant effect
Digoxin	St John's wort	Decreased digoxin levels
	Liquorice	Increased risk of digoxin toxicity via hypokalaemia
Insulin, oral hypoglycaemics	*Panax ginseng*	Hypoglycaemia
Non-steroidal anti-inflammatory drugs (NSAIDs)	Feverfew, garlic (high doses), ginger, ginkgo, ginseng	Decreased platelet aggregation, prolonged bleeding time
Oral contraceptive pill	St John's wort	Reduced efficacy of oral contraceptive pill
Phenothiazine	Evening primrose	Increased risk of provoking fits
Protease inhibitors	Garlic, St John's wort	Reduced blood levels of protease inhibitor (saquinavir with garlic and indinavir with St John's wort)
Spironolactone	Liquorice	Antagonism
Triptans	St John's wort	Lowered blood levels
Warfarin	Danshen, devil's claw	Increased INR
	St John's wort, *Panax ginseng*	Decreased INR
	Feverfew, garlic (high doses), ginger, ginkgo	Decreased platelet aggregation, prolonged bleeding time

Chinese herbal medicine

David Brown

What is it?

Chinese herbal medicine has a different historical basis from European herbalism. It is one component of an ancient and integrated healing art – traditional Chinese medicine (TCM). The other ingredients are acupuncture and exercises such as t'ai chi. The guiding principles of TCM are the flow of life energy, qi, and the balance of the opposing forces of yin and yang. It is estimated that 30–50% of total medicine consumption in China is herbal. Most Chinese herbal medicine (CHM) is used in the form of mixtures of several herbs, formulated to treat an individual's specific imbalance. CHM has become popular in the West (Fig. 40), its appeal lying in it being perceived as ancient, oriental, mystic and wise.

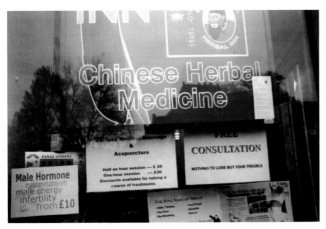

Fig. 40 **Chinese herbal medicine shops are found in many high streets.** (Photograph courtesy of Dr Alistair McKenzie.)

What is the evidence?

There is particular difficulty in obtaining evidence for CHM as the work has been done in Chinese. Few trials have been found which are acceptable in terms of quality, most failing on methodology. Very few showed evidence of long-term benefit (Tang et al 1999).

Safety problems

Many CHMs contain herbs with potent pharmaceutical actions. An example of such a product is *Aristolochia*. The importation, sale or supply of unlicensed medicines containing this or a number of herbs with which it could be confused were prohibited in 2001. This followed two reports of renal failure in the UK linked to use of a herbal slimming aid, Fang Ji. Similar problems had occurred in Europe with Chinese slimming aids. In Belgium 80 women were affected, half of them requiring renal transplantation (Vanherweghem et al 1993, Vanherweghem 1998). The problem was originally attributed to *Stephandria*, but chemical analysis showed that the nephrotoxicity was, in fact, due to *Aristolochia*. The wrong herb had been used in the slimming aid. The name Fang Ji applies to seven different species in Chinese, including *Stephandria tetranda* and *Aristolochia fangchi*.

A product that caused encephalopathy and neuropathy in Hong Kong was supposedly made from a gentian but, in fact, contained *Podophyllum* (Ng et al 1991).

A report from California (Slifman et al 1998) describes two cases of apparent digitalis toxicity in patients not knowingly taking the drug. Both, however, had been using a course of botanical preparations for 'internal cleansing'. One of the products was shown to contain digitalis glycosides. The manufacturer claimed the product only contained plantain. Analysis of the raw material confirmed the presence of *Digitalis lanata*. This was a 6000 lb batch of 'plantain' which had been imported from Germany 2 years previously and had been distributed to 150 manufacturers, distributors and retailers.

Adulteration of CHMs with conventional medicines, presumably to enhance their efficacy, also occurs. The Consumers' Association bought five creams for eczema from five Chinese herbalists and had them analysed. Two contained steroids; one, Bejing Tong Ren Tang, contained five different steroids. Several of the products bought by the Consumers' Association had either no label

or only one in Chinese. Consumers are advised not to purchase products without labels that they understand. Even then, there is no guarantee that the label is accurate.

Tang et al (1999) analysed 11 Chinese herbal creams obtained from patients attending dermatology clinics, and showed that 8 of the 11 contained dexamethasone in concentrations ranging from 64 to 1500 µg/g.

In a study of CHMs in Taiwan (Huang 1997), 24% were found to contain pharmaceutical drugs, the commonest being caffeine, paracetamol, indometacin, diuretics and prednisolone.

In California, heavy metals were found in significant amounts in CHMs (Ko 1998); 243 products were analysed, of which 36 contained arsenic, 24 lead and 35 mercury, all at levels above the legal limits for oral pharmaceuticals. Prescription medicines including chlorpheniramine, testosterone and ephedrine were found in 17 products. In all, 83 products had undeclared pharmaceuticals or heavy metals and 23 had more than one adulterant.

The MHRA list non-herbal ingredients that can be found in CHMs internationally but which should not be sold in UK under the terms of legislation governing herbal products. These are listed as mineral or animal ingredients. Some of these ingredients are restricted under the Convention on International Trade in Endangered Species of Wild Fauna and Flora. Some seem dangerous, e.g. cinnabaris (i.e. mercuric sulphide) and realgar (i.e. arsenic sulphide). Others such as silkworm faeces, testicles and penis of bear, fossilised teeth, squirrel excrement and human placenta may, to some, be aesthetically challenging.

The fact that such substances are listed in a pharmacopoeia abroad does not make them legal in the UK. Products have been claimed to have their formulation modified to exclude non-permitted ingredients from CHMs sold in the UK. Analysis has not shown such assurances to be uniformly reliable.

Sources of further information

- Barnes J, Anderson L, Phillipson D 2002 Herbal medicines: a guide for healthcare professionals, 2nd edn. Pharmaceutical Press, London
- Medicines Control Agency. July 2002. Safety of herbal medicinal products
- Tang J L, Zhan S Y, Ernst E 1999 Review of randomised controlled trials of traditional Chinese medicine. British Medical Journal 319(7203):160–161
- Traditional Herbal Medicine Registration Scheme: guidance and information. Online. Available: www.mhra.gov.uk/home, under 'Safety information', then 'Herbal medicine', then 'Traditional Chinese medicines' June 2005
- World Health Organization Fact Sheet No 134. May 2003. Traditional medicine

---

Key points

- There is no body of evidence to support the claims of efficacy made for Chinese herbal medicines, whether bought in the UK or abroad.
- Chinese herbal medicine may contain herbs with dangerous toxicity, whether bought in the United Kingdom or abroad.
- Chinese herbal medicine may contain contaminants, animal products, minerals or potent conventional drugs.
- Statement of contents on the label may be inaccurate, in Chinese, or absent.

Hypnosis

Alastair Dobbin

What is hypnosis?

Hypnosis is the process of altering mental state by manipulating attention circuitry in the brain, and removing the normal supervisory control of the mind. In this state, access to visualisation, relaxation and problem-solving abilities are improved, and these can be utilised in *hypnotherapy* to alter mood and increase creativity in practical, social and emotional problems. Hypnotherapy can also access repressed memories, allowing manipulation of past traumatic memories to free up the mind from intrusive thoughts or enabling the mind to gain access to positive material it has previously been unable to access.

Hypnosis shares many things in common with the Eastern disciplines of meditation and yoga, both of which facilitate the entry to altered mental state (see 'Mindfulness' box).

Mindfulness

Mindfulness, developed about the same time as yoga 5000 years ago, is a condition in which the student learns to concentrate on internal sensory and cognitive stimuli (breathing, hearing and visualisation), allowing dissociation from or 'letting go' of other stimuli, e.g. sound, anxiety or pain, by inhibition of extraneous neural activity. As well as hypnosis many other therapies share similar mechanisms and techniques for the manipulation of attention such as meditation, autogenic training and yoga.

Some randomised control trials of mind–body therapies have shown positive effects in:

- depression or anxiety (meditation)
- carpal tunnel syndrome (yoga)[a]
- recurrent genital herpes (hypnosis)
- relief of pain in labour (hypnosis)[a]
- back pain (autogenic training)[a]
- asthma (yoga)[a]
- migraine (autogenic training)[a]

[a]In Cochrane Database of Systematic Reviews.

History of hypnosis

In ancient Egypt in the 5th century BC there were 'sleep temples' (temples of healing) which spread in the 4th century to Greece and then to Rome. Modern hypnotism started with the work of Franz Anton Mesmer, who wrote his doctoral thesis on the effects of the magnetic fields of the planets on the human body (1766). He drew heavily on theories of the tides, and the effects of gravity and magnetism on the human body, an extension of Newton's theories. Observing remarkable cures with exorcism, he believed the priest was affecting the sufferers through magnetic fields from his crucifix. Eventually he fell out of favour, fled Vienna and established a school of 'Mesmerism' in Paris. Early French medicine was heavily influenced by hypnosis, and Charcot (1825–1893) held public demonstrations using hypnotism to cure hysterical illness (Fig. 41).

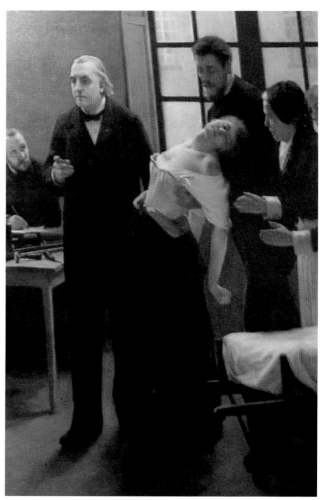

Fig. 41 **Charcot lecturing on hypnosis.**

Freud trained as a hypnotist, as did many doctors in his day, and was apprenticed to Charcot. He was very impressed by Charcot and teamed up with Joseph Breuer in Vienna, curing hysterical paralysis with hypnosis. From his observations of patients under hypnosis, Freud formed his theory of the mind, which is the foundation for all modern psychotherapy. Freud rejected hypnosis for psychoanalysis, which postulates that if you bring unconscious material to the conscious mind you can cure people of any mental disorder. There has never been any empirical evidence for the success of this therapeutic model and it is ironic that a man who cured people with hypnosis developed a technique which by his own admission had little effect, yet is now the basis for modern psychotherapy. The British Medical Association (BMA) and the American Medical Association (AMA) in the 1950s both approved the use of hypnotherapy for the treatment of certain conditions. In 1995, the National Institutes of Health (NIH) assessment panel in the US recommended that hypnosis be considered an effective treatment for chronic pain and recommended that hypnosis patients be reimbursed by insurance companies.

Regulation

All medically qualified doctors are covered to practise hypnosis without any special qualification, although in the course of an enquiry a doctor would need to demonstrate competence to a hypnotising peer. Medical staff and allied professions have their own society dedicated to hypnosis (see Sources of further information) and there is a British peer reviewed journal of hypnosis, *Contemporary Hypnosis*, available on Medline. Doctors usually use hypnosis privately; there are very few family doctors or specialists using hypnosis on their NHS patients. The number of doctors using hypnotherapy is small; most patients will therefore go to a lay hypnotist. There are no formal regulations regarding the training and practice of hypnotherapy; unfortunately neither is there a statutory regulatory body, therefore there are many organisations and training courses.

Dangers of hypnosis

Most hypnotists think it unwise to treat psychotic or suicidal patients. A patient with depression requires assessment for suicidal risks before being treated with hypnosis, otherwise hypnosis is generally regarded as safe. As with all complementary therapies, it is important not to overlook conventional medical diagnosis and treatment.

Role within conventional medicine

Hypnosis can be used in a variety of physical and psychiatric conditions. The conditions it is generally used for are:

- psychiatric: anxiety, depression, phobia, post-traumatic stress, psychosexual disorders
- physical: migraine, tension headache, irritable bowel, chronic pain, functional dyspepsia and vomiting, enuresis, skin problems and cardiac arrhythmias
- habit: smoking, obesity, blushing, nail biting, tics and shyness.

Evidence for its success is variable; although the effects of hypnosis often reach significance in the laboratory, the results from clinical trials are much more variable.

There are many uses of hypnosis and visualisation in conventional medicine. A full induction into a 'trance' is not always necessary, and it can thus be of use in the acute situation to calm a child having a suture or a dressing or a nervous patient having a tooth extraction and in patients experiencing acute anxiety. In its more conventional guise, held over a number of sessions, it can be used in any of the above conditions.

A typical hypnosis session

A hypnosis session may entail the patient being guided into a deeply relaxed state and becoming pain-free physically or emotionally, with suggestions given that the unconscious mind can access a solution to the current problem (Fig. 42). The patient may signal agreement by unconscious movements, and describe past events under hypnosis.

The hypnotist may well 'anchor' a problem-solving relaxed state on a word or an action so that this becomes a 'shortcut'

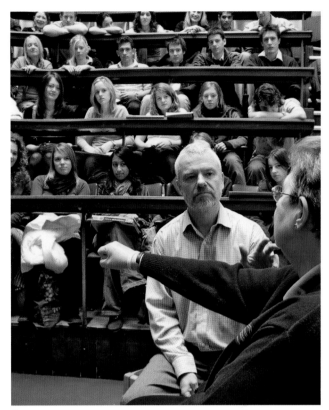

Fig. 42 **GP demonstrating hypnosis to a class of medical students.** (Photograph courtesy of University of Edinburgh).

and the client is subsequently able to access this state easily and effectively. Clients can then practise this 'self-hypnosis' in their everyday existence, which may well flip their mood and allow access to a more solution-based thought process, greatly improving their quality of life. The client may also be given a self-hypnosis CD that may boost the therapeutic effect. Classical hypnosis was reframed in the 1960s in California into the techniques of neurolinguistic programming (NLP). This recognised the common features of a number of successful therapists, among them Milton Erickson, a legendary hypnotist with an ability to transform people with his brand of dialectic linguistics. NLP uses very effective shortcuts, and tends to use the classical trance state less although still dealing with the unconscious (see Sources of further information).

Who can be hypnotised?

The ability to be hypnotised, *susceptibility*, is a stable trait which does not change through a person's life. For some it is easy (high susceptible), for some not at all (low susceptible). Most lie somewhere along the spectrum between. This trait is independent of age, sex, and experience of hypnotist. Hypnosis even in a low susceptible is as effective as placebo in treating pain, and in a high susceptible is three times as effective as placebo (see 'Stop and think' box). Irrespective of susceptibility, an important factor for success is the trust in the hypnotist, and the power of their reputation. This increases the *suggestibility* of the client. General practitioners and anyone practising hypnosis within the NHS, for example nurses or physiotherapists, as trusted members of society, could expect good results.

Hypnosis – is it a special state or psychosocial phenomenon?

In the 20th century Pavlov recognised that neural inhibition was of fundamental importance in the way the brain worked, so that when attending to or responding to one stimulus there will always be reciprocal inhibition of incompatible stimuli and responses. Pavlov recognised that words were conditioned stimuli that could similarly manipulate conscious states to liberate certain areas of the brain. Pavlov was one of the few scientists interested in hypnosis in the early 20th century, and hypnosis can be explained in terms of Pavlovian conditioning (Barrios 2001). In the last 30 years there has been much debate about whether hypnosis is a special 'state' or merely the fulfilment of the client's expectations of hypnosis, i.e. a 'psychosocial' response. In the late 1980s a series of experiments at Imperial College, London, showed specific neurological changes under hypnosis, which the subject could not have imagined or expected; the shifting of mental processing from the left to the right side with changes in specific right-sided functions, such as the ability to sort shapes with the left hand (Gruzelier 1998).

Hypnosis and problem-solving

Positron emission scans (PET) scans show changes in regional cerebral blood flow (rCBF). This has demonstrated that hypnosis is a dynamic process involving shifting activation of different cortical and subcortical regions involving visualisation and problem-solving areas (Rainville et al 1999). The areas of the brain most consistently stimulated by hypnosis are the thalamus, insula, occipital lobes and the anterior cingulate cortex (ACC). The ACC appears to have an important role in monitoring the reward status of the brain's current attentional state and to switch strategies to maintain such a rewarded state. It is developmentally and histologically part of the motor cortex, so it will suggest an alternative strategy or motor 'solution' to any unrewarded state, i.e. to problem solve. Scans show the brain using this same solution 'tool' in both social and physical pain (Eisenberger & Lieberman 2004). Anxiety inhibits the use of this tool, thereby cutting us off from the solution. By dissociating the brain from its anxiety, probably all mind–body techniques allow more effective engagement of problem-solving by this route.

Sources of further information

- Bandler R, Grindler J 1979 Frogs into princes. Real People Press, Utah

- British Autogenic Society (BAS): www.autogenic-therapy.org.uk
- British Society for Medical and Dental Hypnosis (BSMDH): www.bsmdh.com and www.bsmdh-scot.com
- Heap M, Aravind K K (eds) 2001 Hartland's medical and dental hypnosis, 4th edn. Elsevier, Edinburgh
- WholeHealthMD.com: www.wholehealthMD.com. (Good advice on yoga or meditation in reference library)

Case study

Dental phobia: 'classical' hypnosis

A 60-year-old woman had not visited the dentist since her 20s. She thought it was because of a difficult dental extraction aged 5. In trance her unconscious mind was asked if it would go back to the source of the problem. She recalled being out with her father at the swings aged 4, falling off the swing and being concussed. Her father panicked and thought she might be badly injured. She picked up on his fear, and feared that she might die. The hypnotist gave her a visualisation of her adult self helping the child. After the session she said that her conscious mind had completely forgotten the incident until this session. She subsequently visited the dentist many times without fear.

Case study

Migraine: 'modern' NLP treatment

A 40-year-old woman had classical migraines almost every week for 20 years. These were very disabling and frequently resulted in time off work. She visited the doctor and whilst she was in a trance he helped her identify good strong coping feelings. Her unconscious then helped her find the trigger for her migraines and she was then able to overcome this using the coping feelings. She has not had a migraine since.

STOP THINK

- Is suggestion the same as self-hypnosis?
- Placebo has been described as the 'self fulfilling nature of response expectancies'.
- Why is the placebo effect apparently so powerful in some conditions?
- Is the placebo effect that of suggestion and/or visualisation – indeed is there a difference?
- What therapies can legitimately utilise the placebo effect?
- What are mind–body therapies?

Prayer and faith healing

Michael T. Ross and Scott A. Murray

What is prayer?

Prayer can be defined as 'A solemn and humble request to God, or to an object of worship; a supplication, petition, or thanksgiving, usually expressed in words' (Simpson & Weiner 1989). Prayers can be roughly divided into four components – petition (asking for healing, relief of suffering, guidance or strength), thanksgiving (praise for what has been done and in faith for what will be done), confession (admitting sins and seeking forgiveness) and connection (developing union and relationship with God) – although many have aspects of all four.

Faith healing is a collective term for two distinctly different interventions – one a religious faith that prayers for healing will be answered by God; the other is a more humanistic view in which the therapist effects healing. This chapter will focus on some of the key concepts of prayer for healing and religious faith healing from a conventional Western medical perspective with extensive reference to the literature. Many of the principles and examples in this chapter (and in the medical literature) are Christian in origin. However, it is intended to be accessible to those of different faiths or with no religious background.

Background

Monasteries were the seat of conventional medical knowledge and practice in medieval Europe until the early 13th century (Loudon 1997). Many healthcare professionals believe their faith is very important to their work. Others, however, are wary of religion – not least because of historical religious bigotry and self-promoting 'television evangelists' (Barrett 2003). Whatever our own beliefs, a recent study of CAM use in 31,044 US adults found 45% had in the past year used some form of prayer for healing compared to 36% using all other CAM (Barnes et al 2004). The Cochrane complementary medicine field now contains 'prayer' and 'faith healing' topics (Cochrane Collaboration 2005) and they have already completed a review of intercessory prayer (Fig. 43).

Seventy-six per cent of the British population feel there is a spiritual dimension to their lives (Hay & Hunt 2000) and interest increases when people are faced with life-threatening illness (Lo et al 2002). Recent studies found that 85% of physicians thought they should be aware of patients' spirituality, although less than half of these felt they should enquire routinely (Monroe et al 2003). Seventy-seven per cent of inpatients believed their physicians should consider their spiritual beliefs (King & Bushwick 1994).

Christians, Jews, Muslims, Hindi and many others pray to God(s) for healing. Sometimes their religion specifically encourages this, as in the Muslim and Christian faiths:

> Pray for each other so that you may be healed
> (James 5:13 NIV).

Buddhist, New Age, Pagan, First Nation American people and others also pray for healing, although not always to God(s) as such. None of these faiths claim that the praying individuals themselves have the power to heal, rather they appeal to God(s) or another 'object of worship' to effect the healing, based on several assumptions (Table 19). This key factor differentiates prayer and religious faith healing from cognitive therapy, reiki, therapeutic touch, magic, spiritual healing and the humanist 'mind-over-matter' faith healing.

How do people pray?

(See the case studies 'Remote intercessory prayer' and 'Retroactive intercessory prayer'.)

Many different types of prayer are reported in the medical literature (Table 20). Religions and individuals have diverse approaches to prayer and stress the importance of different

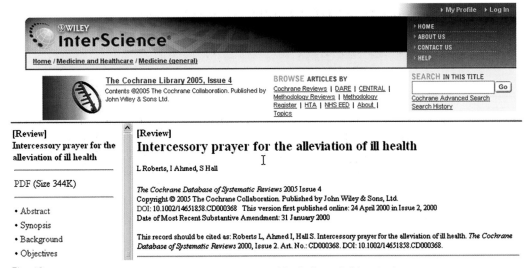

Fig. 43 **Cochrane report on intercessory prayer.** (Courtesy of the Cochrane Collaboration.)

Table 19 Basic assumptions in prayers for healing

- God(s) or another supernatural force exists
- Illness is undesirable (although may have positive outcomes)
- God can heal illness and relieve suffering
- God will hear requests for healing
- God may act on such requests

Table 20 Types of prayer for healing in the medical literature

1. Praying for oneself
2. Praying for each other in a group
3. Praying for others
   (a) In their presence – 'local intercessory prayer'
   (b) Involving touch such as 'laying-on of hands'
   (c) At a distance – 'remote intercessory prayer' (see case study)
   (d) For past events – 'retroactive intercessory prayer' which assume God is not constrained by linear time (see case study)
4. Praying for the 'intercessors' that are praying for others

aspects such as fasting, facing towards Mecca, putting the hands together (Fig. 44), playing music or dancing, adopting a yoga position or the wearing of talismans and amulets (Rosner 1999). These stereotypical actions are by no means universal, however – many people pray whilst doing everyday activities such as walking, driving or housework.

Some prayers consist of repetitive phrases with religious significance such as the Catholic 'rosary', Buddhist 'mantra', or Muslim 'ruqya' (healing prayers, during which the right hand is passed over the painful area). Many prayers are more spontaneous and sound more like a conversation or a stream of consciousness that can be spoken, thought silently, written down or voiced in another medium such as song or dance. Some prayers are not voiced at all but rather involve stillness and 'waiting on God' (Cooke 2003). Many prayers ask 'thy will be done' for the best outcome or for healing generally whilst others ask for specific therapeutic outcomes (McCaffrey et al 2004, Dossey 1993).

Mechanisms of prayer for healing and evidence

A common religious objection to the scientific study of prayer is that it seems heretical – questioning the very existence or power of God. Others believe there are natural laws we do not yet understand in prayer and faith healing that may be amenable to scientific study. It was once thought heretical to suggest the Earth was round and orbited the

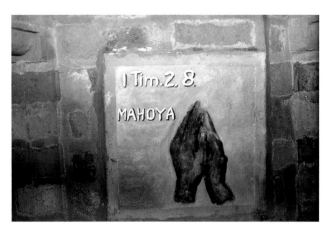

Fig. 44 **Praying hands on the wall of a hospital chapel in Chogoria, Kenya.** (Photograph courtesy of Professor Scott A. Murray.)

sun. Our position is that an evidence-based approach to prayer is not a way of trying to prove God exists or even prove God answers prayers, but is simply a study of prayer as a healthcare intervention:

> Using the rules of one theory to test the other is almost bound to make it look nonsense. It would, to take a hackneyed example, be pointless to investigate the existence of God by a controlled trial of the efficacy of prayer. (Martyn 1995)

Research in this area has been of variable quality. However, we have identified in the medical literature five thematic mechanisms by which prayer and faith for healing could have effects.

1. Individual biological and psychological effects of praying

Prayer and religious commitment have been associated with increased longevity and beneficial biological and psychological effects such as relaxation, reduced depression and substance abuse, reduced blood pressure, better coping with illness and better recovery after operation (Matthews et al 1998). Specific practices such as the Catholic rosary or yoga mantras have also been shown to enhance heart rate variability and baroreflex sensitivity, which are associated with improved prognosis in cardiovascular disease (Bernardi et al 2001).

2. Social aspects of prayer and religion

The relationship between social factors and health is long established. Church attendance and other religious activities have been associated with better physical and mental health in many different studies (Koenig 2000), although this may in part be confounded by other factors such as age, race, socio-economic status and lower use of alcohol and tobacco (Sloan et al 1999).

3. Placebo effect

As discussed in Section 3, the placebo effect of any CAM can be very significant. Individuals who pray and those who know they are being prayed for are also likely to derive benefit from the placebo effect, which may be enhanced by the context of the prayers and by social pressures (Barrett 2003).

4. The effects of positive thinking on others

A meta-analysis of 832 studies has demonstrated that random events (such as number generators and radioactive decay) can be influenced by human thought alone (Radin & Nelson 1989). Experiments on mental influence on bacterial and fungal growth, human biochemical processes and tissues and a variety of other subjects have repeatedly demonstrated that visualisation and 'intentionality' can have an external influence (Dossey 1993, 2004).

5. Divine responses to prayer

Many religions believe God usually responds to prayer and heals through healthcare professionals and in other 'natural' ways:

> [God] can bring healing without medicine, and does so at times, but normally works through the doctors … do not imagine that it is somehow holier to be healed through prayer than through antibiotics. The same God is at work through both (Green 1998).

However, most also believe that God may also heal illness by 'miracle' (apparently supernatural events which cannot be explained by current scientific knowledge).

> As a physician, I have seen men, after all other therapy has failed, lifted out of disease and melancholy by the serene effort of prayer. It is the only power in the world that seems to overcome the so-called 'laws of nature'. (Alexis Carrel, in Woodard 1959)

There are innumerable case reports from sacred, secular and medical literature suggesting that miracles have happened in the past and are still occurring (e.g. Cooke 2003, Rosner 1999, Woodard 1959). Believers emphasise the importance of faith, deeper knowledge and personal experience in appreciating and recognising divine intervention. They may argue that the study of prayer is confounded by a lack of control groups free from 'background' prayer or separated from God's influence, and that God does not respond in measurable dose–response curves (Myers 2000). Sceptics suggest 'miracles' are coincidence, providence and errors in diagnosis or reporting. Many recent scientific studies have shown a positive effect of prayer on health, although others looking at smoking cessation, leukaemia, AIDS and heart disease have shown no significant benefit. A recent comprehensive Cochrane review entitled 'Intercessory prayer for the alleviation of ill health' concluded 'If prayer is seen as a human endeavour it may or may not be beneficial and further trials could uncover this … if any benefit derives from God's response to prayer it may be beyond any such trials to prove or disprove' (Roberts et al 2000; Fig. 43).

Potential harmful effects of prayer

Prayer is typically used in addition to conventional medicine, although some may use it as an alternative on occasion. Less common are individuals or even whole communities who consistently rely on prayer for healing. Christian Scientists, for example, reject conventional medicine and have developed entirely prayer-based approaches to healthcare, fees for which can be claimed from Medicare or as tax-exempt medical expenses in the US. In some American states there are even religious exemptions from child neglect laws obliging parents to seek medical care for seriously ill children (Simpson 1989). A study of child deaths from 1975 to 1995 found 172 cases where the documented histories suggest a failure to seek medical care due to over-reliance on faith healing (Asser & Swan 1998). Of these children, 140 had conditions for which survival with medical care could have exceeded 90% such as birth asphyxia, pneumonia, diabetes, appendicitis, dehydration and meningitis. It was not possible in that study to compare incidence or mortality rates with the general population as there are an unknown number of people rejecting conventional medicine on religious grounds, but the authors conclude that most of the deaths could have been prevented.

Some individuals blame themselves for their illness or failure to be healed (Murray et al 2004), and may even be told by others that their lack of healing is due to sin or insufficient faith. There are also concerns that patients may not come to terms with the fact that they are dying because of a false hope that they will be healed, or may believe they have been healed when they have not (Barrett 2003).

In a 1994 Gallup poll 5% of Americans admitted to praying that harm would come to others, and many traditional cultures have 'prayers', hexes and curses for harm. Several researchers have observed that bacterial and fungal growth can be inhibited by 'prayer' and conscious thought, and suggest that negative 'prayers' or 'hexes' may indeed cause harm (Dossey 2004). Even if one believes God could not be influenced to effect a negative outcome, if there are remote effects of conscious thought which are not related to divine intervention, as Dossey suggests, one would predict these could be negative as well as positive.

The role of prayer within conventional medicine

Most doctors agree they should not try to influence patients' religious beliefs (Table 21). The UK General Medical Council (GMC) has stated that doctors have a duty to 'Make sure that your personal beliefs do not prejudice your patients' care' and 'Avoid abusing your position as a doctor' (GMC 2001). Other particularly relevant ethico-legal issues are confidentiality (sharing clinical information to help people pray for an individual), consent (is it acceptable to pray for anyone without consent?) and equality (should one only pray for people of the same religion?). Religious healthcare professionals may also have to consider their own religious ethics – for example, if their religion tells them to pray for the sick, is it ever right to know about people who are sick without praying for them? It may be difficult to know when to pray and when not to, who and what to pray for and even where to pray, as there are not always suitable locations in healthcare settings (Sheikh 1997).

In a recent American survey, only 11% of those praying for health concerns had discussed this with their physicians (McCaffrey et al 2004), yet many doctors recognise the benefits of exploring spiritual issues with patients (Monroe et al 2003). Hospital chaplaincy is increasingly available. However, it may not address the needs of a multi-faith society (Gatrad et al 2003) and some patients may prefer to discuss such issues with healthcare professionals. Holistic quality of life instruments also now include the spiritual domain (WHO 1998) and some principles have been proposed to facilitate the exploration of a patient's spiritual beliefs without compromising the health professional's responsibilities (Koenig 2000; Table 22). Not all patients who mention they are religious or have been praying want their doctor to explore these issues in detail, and indeed this may not be appropriate. However, being aware of these aspects of a patient's life can enhance understanding and develop the doctor–patient relationship.

Table 21 **Guiding principles for medical practitioners**
Physicians should not:
1. 'Prescribe' religious beliefs or activities for health reasons
2. Impose religious beliefs or initiate prayer without knowledge of the patient's religious background
3. Provide in-depth religious counselling
4. Pray with a patient without his or her explicit request (and only if this is the preference of the patient or no religious professional is available)
Physicians should:
1. Acknowledge and respect the spiritual lives of patients, which may involve taking a 'spiritual history' (Table 22)
2. Consider supporting the patient's religious beliefs that aid coping with illness

Adapted from Koenig (2000).

Case study

Remote intercessory prayer

In one double-blind study, 393 consenting patients admitted to a coronary care unit (CCU) were randomly divided into two similar groups, one of which was the object of remote Christian prayer from 3–7 'intercessors' during their stay. The prayer group had overall better outcomes, and had lower incidence of cardiopulmonary arrest (2% versus 7%) and intubation/ventilation (0% versus 6%); pneumonia (3% versus 13%) and antibiotics (2% versus 9%); congestive cardiac failure (8% versus 20%) and diuretics (3% versus 8%). There was no statistically significant difference in mortality (7% versus 9%) or days spent in hospital (Byrd 1988). A similar double-blind study involving 1013 CCU patients also found that the prayer group had significantly less overall morbidity (11% reduction in weighted outcome scores), but had similar mortality and duration of stay to the control group (Harris et al 1999).

Summary

- Spiritual issues may be important to patients and they may wish to discuss these with their doctor.
- Prayers for healing and faith healing are very common, are practised by many different religions and are very significant for many people.
- Prayer is a common response to the existential angst which is periodically part of the human condition.
- Various types of prayer have been studied in a scientific manner with a number of positive results, although a recent Cochrane review did not find conclusive evidence.

- Several contributing mechanisms have been suggested for the effectiveness of prayer, some of which may be biological.
- Prayer may also have harmful effects, and care and sensitivity are required for physicians to respond appropriately to the spiritual needs of their patients.

Table 22 **Sample questions for taking a simple spiritual history (Lo et al 1999)**

- Is faith (religion, spirituality) important to you in this illness?
- Has faith (religion, spirituality) been important to you at other times in your life?
- Do you have someone to talk to about religious matters?
- Would you like to explore religious matters with someone?

Case study

Retroactive intercessory prayer

A total of 3393 septicaemic patients known to have been patients in an Israeli hospital between 1990 and 1996 were randomly divided into two similar groups several years later. One individual said 'a short prayer' for the intervention group without knowing what their clinical outcome had been. When subsequently comparing outcomes, the number of days of fever and days in hospital was significantly lower in the intervention group than the control. The small reduction in mortality did not reach statistical significance (Leibovici 2001).

STOP THINK A patient asks 'Could you pray with me?' 'Doctor, are you religious? Do you believe in God?'

Acupuncture

Marie Fallon and Karen R. Simpson

What is it?

Acupuncture is seen as a therapeutic and preventative practice that aims to manage a variety of disorders and complaints (Fig. 45). It involves the practice of inserting fine needles under the skin and underlying tissues in specific points of the body to stimulate nerve impulses.

It is one of the most popular CAM therapies used by people in the Western world and is seen by many conventional practitioners as an acceptable CAM therapy (Lipman et al 2003).

History

Acupuncture is one of the oldest forms of medicine recorded. However, the exact origin is unclear with reports that it may have been as early as the 21st century BC (Ma 1992). Towards the end of the 17th century, Dr Willhelm Ten Rhyne, a physician employed by the Dutch East India

Company and stationed in Japan, introduced it into Europe. The therapy lost popularity and professional interest in the West in the 1800s. In Britain, the study of traditional acupuncture did not develop again until the 1950s and early 1960s. In 1972, an American journalist, James Reston, travelling with President Nixon had his appendix removed and benefited from acupuncture analgesia postoperatively. President Nixon was so impressed that he helped to organise a cultural exchange of medical practitioners between the US and China. Later that same year, thirty acupuncturists from China were invited to participate in a programme at the University of California, Los Angeles Medical School. As a result acupuncture was reintroduced into conventional medicine.

Types of acupuncture

There are two main types of acupuncture. The traditional Eastern style involves a sophisticated and elaborate system

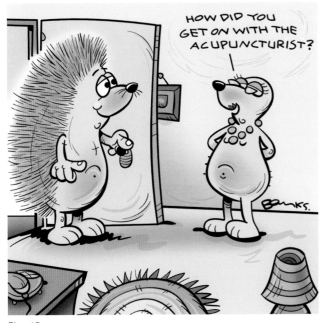

Fig. 45

Table 23 **Acupuncture techniques and variations**	
Traditional Chinese acupuncture	'Qi' or energetic system with flow of vital energy
	Yin and yang need to be balanced in health
	Pulse and tongue diagnosis and several laws utilised for traditional diagnosis
	'De qi' or needling sensation elicited with vigorous stimulation up to 30 min ± moxibustion
Western acupuncture	Manual acupuncture
	Minimal stimulation up to 20 min
	Maximal stimulation intermittently up to 20 min
	Electroacupuncture
	2–4 Hz low frequency
	50–200 Hz high frequency
Acupuncture analgesia	Vigorous manual stimulation or electroacupuncture
	Used for operations in China now as sole anaesthetic in approximately 6% of operations
Acupressure	No needles – less effective than needling
Auricular acupuncture	Needles inserted into tender regions or 'recipe' points
Cupping	Place warmed cups on specific acupuncture points to bring blood and energy to the surface
Ryodoraku	Reduced skin impedance treated electrically
Laser therapy	No needles – advantageous in paediatrics (not strictly acupuncture)
Veterinary	± electroacupuncture, unlikely to be a placebo

of diagnosis based on 'energy flow' round the body, with subsequent selection of acupuncture points for stimulation by the insertion of fine needles in order to effect a 'cure'. Western practitioners use acupuncture following orthodox Western diagnosis by history, examination and special investigations initially, and use either a traditional form of acupuncture or a simplified neurophysiologically based method of point selection. There are various acupuncture techniques currently available (Table 23).

Regulation and training

There is no current legislation covering acupuncture in Britain. However, the Department of Health is proposing to publish regulations under Section 60 of the Health Act 1999. This means that acupuncture practitioners can currently register with a number of organisations, and there is no single list of acupuncturists in the UK that the public can access. Over 2000 acupuncturists are registered with the British Acupuncture Council.

The British Acupuncture Council (BAcC) was formed in 1995 and is the largest single organisation. It is an amalgamation of five separate organisations, who agreed that one body should represent and govern their professionally qualified traditional acupuncturists in all aspects of their work. Nevertheless, there is no statutory regulation for acupuncturists to be registered.

The BAcC does have common standards of education, ethics, discipline and codes of practice to ensure the health and safety of the public at all times. Members carry insurance in the same way as doctors do. The training of member acupuncturists is regulated by the British Acupuncture Accreditation Board, and is for a minimum of 2 years full time or its equivalent on a part-time basis. However, there is no single national recognised core curriculum. A variety of acupuncture training courses are available from short courses to Masters courses, including undergraduate modules and degrees as well as short or long postgraduate courses.

Role within conventional medicine

Mills & Budd (2000) reported that there are over 3530 statutory health professionals registered with various acupuncture organisations in the UK. There are some general practices, hospitals and special areas offering acupuncture. In addition, there is a call from the public and various organisations to consider making acupuncture more readily available to NHS patients, especially for back and dental pain, migraine headaches, nausea and vomiting. The Department of Health in 1999 reported that it was widely used to treat chronic pain. It is available in approximately 86% of NHS chronic pain services with a limited number of physiotherapists, nurses and clinicians trained in acupuncture (BMA 2000).

Evidence and efficacy issues

The results of clinical trials of acupuncture have been conflicting. This has been partly due to the complex issues surrounding the methodology of acupuncture trials.

Recently 'placebo' acupuncture needles have been used. However, this remains a challenging area of research. Placebo analgesia works in part via stimulation of endogenous opioids, as does acupuncture, so it is quite testing to delineate one effect from the other. This means that key research challenges remain for acupuncture.

Neurotransmitters and clinical effects

There is now strong evidence that many of the analgesic and other effects of acupuncture are due to the action it has on various neurotransmitters (Table 24). Hence the underlying pathophysiology may dictate the optimum regimen for a patient, especially in cases of cancer-induced symptoms.

There is evidence from published trials that acupuncture is more effective than control interventions for back pain, postoperative nausea and vomiting, dental pain and migraines (Melchart et al 2005, Lee & Done 1999, Manheimer et al

Table 24 Clinical effects produced by the action of acupuncture on neurotransmitters

Neurotransmitter system	Action of acupuncture (ACU)	Clinical effects of ACU	Source
5-Hydroxytryptamine (5-HT), serotonin	Stimulates the release of this 5-HT agonist which acts centrally and peripherally via descending pain inhibitory pathways	Analgesia and elevation of mood	Han & Terenius (1982)
Noradrenaline as transmitter in sympathetic nervous system	Stimulates the hypothalamus to activate the efferent sympathetic pathways and so causes the release of this alpha-receptor agonist from postganglionic adrenergic nerve endings	Circulatory and metabolic effects; normalises blood flow and skin temperature	Ernst & Lee (1985); Lundeberg, (1999)
Beta-endorphin	μ opioid agonist (MOR) released preferentially by low-frequency (2 Hz) electroacupuncture	Analgesia. Action blocked by naloxone	Han & Sun (1990); Han et al (1991)
Orphanin OFQ, nociceptin	An opioid which acts at a receptor LC132/ORL1 as an agonist but antagonises the action of morphine. Role not clear, but may operate as a modulator of opioid systems	Analgesic effects of acupuncture may be antagonised by orphanin	Tian et al (1997)
Adrenocorticotrophic hormone (ACTH)	Co-released with beta-endorphin (see above)	Anti-inflammatory, modulates stress, and immune responses	Roth et al (1997)
Cholecystokinin (CCK) and angiotensin (AII)	Stimulates release of CCK and AII which acts as endogenous opioid antagonist	CCK and AII may contribute to the development of tolerance to acupuncture (and possibly opioids)	Zhou et al (1993) Wang & Han (1990)
Gamma-aminobutyric acid (GABA)	TENS releases the inhibitory neurotransmitter GABA from endings of GABA-ergic neurons. Produces presynaptic inhibition of C fibre endings, thereby blocking nociceptive transmission	Segmental analgesia	Garrison & Foreman (1994)
Pre-prometenkephalin, pre-prodynorphin (opioid precursors)	Electroacupuncture (EA) modulates mRNA molecules coding for opioid precursors. EA 2 Hz induces the expression of pre-prodynorphin. Thus, EA may increase the distribution and amount of opioid peptides	This may be one of the mechanisms by which acupuncture induces analgesia of long duration	Guo et al (1996)

2005). On the other hand, there is little to support the belief it works for weight loss, smoking cessation, recovery from stroke, osteoarthritis or tension headaches.

Complications and contraindications

In the hands of properly trained practitioners, acupuncture is safe with a low incidence of side effects. It is certainly safer than many conventional treatments or drugs used. However, any procedure that involves inserting needles into the body has some potential problems (Ernst & White 1997). The adverse effects of acupuncture have been classified into four groups:

- delayed or missed diagnosis of the condition treated
- negative reactions, for example syncope, vertigo and sweating
- bacterial and viral infections (hepatitis B, C and HIV)
- trauma of tissues and organs (rare).

Table 25 lists some contraindications and cautions when doing acupuncture on patients.

Table 25 Some contraindications and precautions

- Do not treat around unstable spine – could potentially lead to spinal cord injury or transection
- Do not directly needle superficial tumour nodules or ulceration
- Do not needle if blood clotting is seriously impaired
- Do not directly needle too close to or into a prosthesis
- Do not use electroacupuncture in a patient with a pacemaker
- Cancer patients can be more sensitive to acupuncture and nursing assistance is recommended for each case
- Needle only very superficially in cachectic patients
- If tolerance occurs – it may represent progressive disease and full investigations of tumour status may be required

Cautions for semi-permanent needles

- Avoid in patients with heart valvular disease, post-heart transplant, or with a pacemaker
- Caution in immunocompromised patients secondary to any cause including chemotherapy and radiotherapy and intensive therapy unit
- Severe immunosuppression
- Post-splenectomy
- Avoid in patients with known hepatitis B or C as risk from needlestick injury if they accidentally 'fall out'
- Strong reactors'

Sources of further information

- Acupuncture Association of Chartered Physiotherapy: http://www.aacp.uk.com/
- Bivins R 2000 Acupuncture: expertise and cross cultural medicine. Palgrave, Manchester
- British Acupuncture Council: http://www.acupuncture.org.uk/
- British Medical Acupuncture Society: http://www.medical-acupuncture.co.uk/

Case study

A typical consultation with an acupuncturist

Before the treatment, the practitioner usually takes a full history including medical and family, lifestyle and diet. A traditional pulse reading is also taken at both wrists followed by clinical observation of the face and tongue to determine the nature of the disharmony. A diagnosis is made and specific points are needled. The needles are left in place for 20 to 30 minutes during which a pleasant sensation is often felt (Fig. 46).

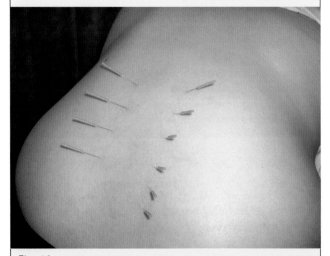

Fig. 46 **Possible position of needles for a client with back pain.** (Courtesy of University of Edinburgh.)

- NHS Direct (acupuncture): http://www.nhsdirect.nhs.uk/
  en.aspx?articleID=6
- Kaptchuk T J 2002 Acupuncture: theory, efficacy and
  practice. Annals of Internal Medicine 136(5):374–383
- Prince of Wales Foundation for Integrated Health:
  http://www.fihealth.org.uk/

STOP THINK

- Should there be one regulatory body
  that requires statutory registration of
  all acupuncturists?
- Has there recently been any 'gold standard'
  research into medical conditions that shows
  that it can be treated effectively by acupuncture?
- Should there be a standardised core
  curriculum for acupuncture that is subject to
  external validation and examination board?
- Should universities provide accredited
  postgraduate courses in acupuncture?

Homeopathy

Thomas E. Whitmarsh

What is homeopathy?

A dictionary definition would be that homeopathy is 'a
therapeutic method using preparations of substances whose
effects when administered to healthy people correspond to
the manifestations of the disorder (symptoms, clinical signs,
pathological states) in the individual patient' (Swayne 2000).
This was expressed by the originator of the method,
Dr Samuel Hahnemann (1755–1843), in the Latin phrase
similia similibus curentur (let like be cured by like) and is
the fundamental principle of homeopathy, the *similia
principle*. The well-known use of extremely dilute medicines
is often supposed to be essential, but in fact it is the mode
of prescription according to the similia principle which
defines homeopathy.

Hahnemann was a medical doctor, trained in the
prevailing practices of late 18th century Europe, which on
the whole relied on heroic treatments with bleeding,
purging and drugging with mixtures of multiple toxic
ingredients, including heavy metals and poisonous plants.
He rebelled against these techniques and resigned himself
to giving up practice and living by translation work. It was
while translating a treatise on materia medica by William
Cullen, a renowned Scottish physician, that he strongly
disagreed with the explanation given for the action of
Peruvian bark (*Cinchona*, containing quinine) in marsh fever
(or malaria). He took some himself and found that he
developed symptoms which he recognised as being very
similar to those of the fever. Thus he developed the similia
principle, the idea that a medicine which causes certain
symptoms in the healthy can cure those symptoms when
encountered in the sick.

Hahnemann was amongst the first to accurately record
the effects on the human organism of medicinal substances
in his experiments on healthy subjects (which he called
provings). He used substances in common medicinal use at
the time (thus mercury, arsenic and belladonna were
amongst materials he made provings of), but recorded their
individual effects rather than as part of multiple mixtures.

He also collected reports of inadvertent poisoning symptoms
from a wide range of materials and, later, was able to add
'cured symptoms' after prescriptions made on homeopathic
principles to build up 'drug pictures' for many substances.
These long lists of symptoms which have been associated
with a substance make up the homeopathic materia medica.
Many provings have been performed since Hahnemann and
many cured symptoms have been added. There are now
over 2500 homeopathic medicines described in various degrees
of detail in materia medicas.

Role of a homeopathic physician

The job of the homeopathic physician is thus to discover
which of these medicines gives the 'best fit' for the sick
individual according to the similia principle. The deeper the
individualised understanding of a person's symptoms and
the way they habitually relate with the world, the better can
be the fit of the selected remedy and the higher the chances
of a beneficial effect of the treatment. This process can
extend well beyond the physical bodily symptoms to include
general characteristics of the organism, such as reactions to
temperature and food preferences, along with psychological
features, such as jealousy or grief. It is in some ways an
analogical process, comparing how a substance exists in
relation to the environment with how an individual manages
this relationship and using the similia principle to hypothesise
a potentially curative prescription.

Use of highly dilute drugs

The contentious issue of the use of very highly dilute drugs
in homeopathy dates from Hahnemann's observation that
when he reduced the dose of his medicines to reduce their
adverse effects in material doses, as long as he followed his
method of vigorous shaking between each dilution step
('succussion'), the therapeutic power of the medicines increased.

Thus homeopathic remedies are prepared from extracts of (usually) naturally occurring substances, which are diluted in stepwise fashion to achieve the required strength, or 'potency' (Fig. 47). Two scales of dilution are commonly employed, the decimal (X) scale and the centesimal scale (C), with dilution factors at each stage of 1:10, or 1:100. Homeopathic remedies are described by the name of the source followed by an indication of which scale of dilution has been used and how many steps of dilution have been made, for example belladonna 30C. In this example, belladonna extract has been diluted 1:100 in sequential steps with succussion between them 30 times. At each stage, 1 drop of the liquid is put into 99 drops of water and shaken, so that the final conventional concentration of the 30C potency is around 10^{-60}, a value so low that there is very little chance of there being any molecules of active drug left in the remedy potency. Homeopaths commonly use remedies at even higher dilutions and the apparent clinical effectiveness of these has led to speculation about the possible role of the prepared solvent in the healing process, with talk of the 'memory of water'.

Role and scope of use

Homeopathy can add to the care of people suffering from a very wide range of problems, from over-the-counter purchase of remedies for simple common ailments, to multilayered, complicated physical and psychological distress (Boyd 1989). For example, in the homeopathic hospitals, it has found a niche in helping symptom management in terminal care and in chronic neurological problems such as multiple sclerosis. It is especially useful to be able to call upon homeopathic expertise for the large number of people suffering from conditions which are poorly defined and for which there are no effective conventional treatments, such as abnormal grief reactions, chronic fatigue states or severe premenstrual syndrome, to name but a few. It is not, of course, a substitute for necessary replacement therapy such as insulin or thyroxine, but even in diabetes or hypothyroidism, homeopathy will have something to add to the well-being of the patient.

Who practises homeopathy? Regulation

Homeopathy is one of the 'big five' CAM therapies identified by the House of Lords Select Committee. Along with acupuncture, osteopathy, chiropractic and herbal medicine, it has the potential to be a complete system of medicine, rather than only a 'bolt on extra' CAM therapy. It has a very unusual theoretical base, yet is very popular and through the UK homeopathic hospitals (Fig. 48) (in Glasgow, London, Bristol, Liverpool and Tunbridge Wells), is the best example of CAM being practised long term within the NHS. In fact the hospitals were incorporated into the NHS from the foundation of the service in 1948 through the Faculty of Homeopathy Act of Parliament. The Faculty of Homeopathy is a registering body which only allows medical professionals to sit its examinations, so homeopathically trained physicians have long experience in and much to say about the benefits of bringing together a high standard of conventional care with a high standard of a CAM system. Regulation of practitioners on the Faculty lists is through their medical regulating body (such as the GMC or GDC (General Dental Council)). The hospitals are staffed by physicians with dual training in medicine and homeopathy. Many GPs have trained in the basics of homeopathic method through Faculty-accredited courses and use homeopathy in their day-to-day work in primary care and may consult privately too. There are a number of Faculty-accredited doctors practising solely as private homeopathic physicians. In addition, there are many non-medically qualified practitioner (NMQP) registering organisations, whose members practise generally outwith the NHS and are voluntarily self-regulated.

Difficulties with homeopathy and evidence in its support

The two main stumbling blocks to the wider acceptance of homeopathy in medicine are the similia principle, treating like with like, which runs against prevailing principles of pharmacology, and the claim for the effectiveness of ultra-molecular dilutions, which seems frankly impossible in our current state of knowledge.

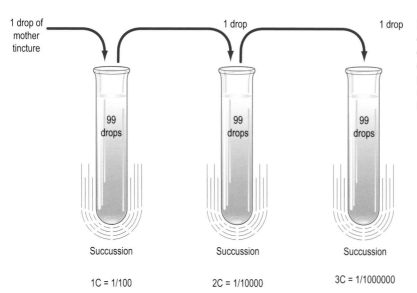

1 drop of mother tincture

1 drop

1 drop

99 drops

99 drops

99 drops

Succussion

Succussion

Succussion

1C = 1/100

2C = 1/10000

3C = 1/1000000

Fig. 47 **Preparing a homeopathic medicine in the centesimal (C) potency scale by the method of serial dilution and succussion.** The process is commonly continued for many more steps to produce, for example, potencies of 6C, 30C and 200C which are then used to medicate granules or tablets of lactose and produce the homeopathic remedy.

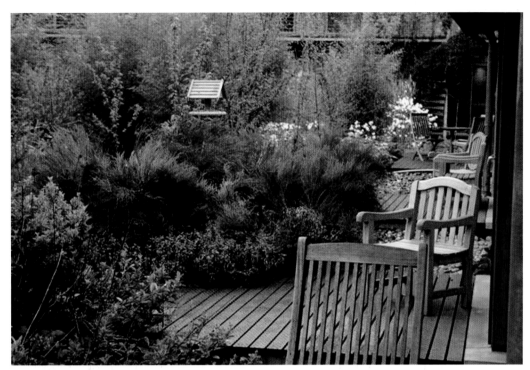

Fig. 48 **Glasgow Homeopathic Hospital (Scotland, UK).** (Photograph courtesy of Jane Kelly.)

In fact, there are many examples from conventional medicine of inadvertent homeopathic uses of drugs. Digoxin in toxic doses causes the arrhythmia which it successfully treats in lower doses. Poisoning with aspirin, an antipyretic, can cause hyperthermia. There are a large number of these seemingly paradoxical effects of well-known conventional drugs (Eskinazi 1999).

Examples exist from biomedical research of biological activity of such things as leukotrienes or tumour necrosis factor (TNF), at concentrations as low as 10^{-19} mol/l (Eskinazi 1999). A recent study showed activity of histamine in submolecular concentrations on the degranulation of basophils (Belon et al 2004). A large body of evidence from across the whole spectrum of biological research has demonstrated non-linear responses to toxic agents, with paradoxical stimulation at low doses, followed by inhibition at higher doses (hormesis) (Calabrese & Baldwin 1998).

For some commentators, no amount of evidence will convince that the effects of homeopathy can be anything more than placebo responses, a function of long consultation times and empathetic listening needed to gain deep understanding of the patient's predicament (Vandenbroucke 1997). Others will point to the double-blind, placebo-controlled trials and their various meta-analyses (Linde et al 1997, Cucherat et al 2000, Mathie 2003) which do support the effectiveness of homeopathy as a therapeutic approach for a wide range of clinical problems.

The small amount of randomised control trials (RCT) research in homeopathy is often bemoaned. This is largely due to lack of funding and a research infrastructure, unsupported as it is by the pharmaceutical industry. There is also a feeling that RCTs are not the best way to show the health benefits of homeopathy. Looking at a clinical area that has been rather better studied than most, migraine and headache, there are at least four RCTs of homeopathy against placebo. One is very positive for homeopathy (Brigo & Serpelloni 1991), two are equivocal (Straumsheim et al 2000, Whitmarsh et al 1997) and one is entirely negative

(Walach et al 1997). A more recent study of real life outcome in a group of headache patients treated homeopathically showed significant improvements in measures of quality of life, which much more closely reflected physicians' and patients' experiences (Muscari-Tomaioli et al 2001). This sort of thinking calls into question the applicability of strict RCT study designs in homeopathy and other CAM therapies (Walach et al 2002).

Safety

There are no direct interactions known between homeopathy and any other medications. Some practitioners have theoretical caution about prescribing remedies made from toxic agents

STOP THINK

- What would be needed for sceptical followers of evidence-based practice to be convinced of the value of homeopathy?
- What would be needed for practitioners of homeopathy to stop using it as they become unconvinced of its value?

Key points

- Homeopathic medicine has a very broad range of clinical applications, including in the many areas in which there is no effective conventional treatment.
- There is accumulating evidence that the response to homeopathic remedies is more than 'just placebo'.
- Learning about homeopathic medicine is a rewarding addition to the clinical skills of any healthcare practitioner.

in pregnancy, but generally one of the major benefits of homeopathy is the possibility to use it in situations where conventional drugs are relatively contraindicated, such as in pregnancy, in the elderly and in children. Any risk on the whole will be indirect, through missed diagnosis or mistaken withholding of necessary conventional treatment by inadequately trained non-medical practitioners.

Sources of further information

- Faculty of Homeopathy (the accrediting and registering body in UK for doctors and other healthcare practitioners): www.trusthomeopathy.org
- Swayne J 1998 Homeopathic method: implications for clinical practice and medical science. Churchill Livingstone, Edinburgh

Massage and aromatherapy

Janet Skinner

The popularity of massage and aromatherapy has increased over the years in Western society. It is offered in the high street, doctors' surgeries, hospitals and privately in individuals' homes and at the workplace.

What is massage and aromatherapy?

Massage therapies involve the use of the hands to perform manipulation of soft tissues by pressure, traction, rubbing or pressing as shown in Figure 49. Aromatherapy is the use of the extract of plant essences in the form of essential oils (Fig. 50) for therapeutic purposes. Essential oils are normally extracted from plants by steam distillation. Aromatherapy massages utilise essential oils to aid the process (Vickers & Zollman 1999). Both of these therapies have been classified as Group 2 therapies by the House of Lords Select Committee report (2000).

History

Massage has been used for many centuries, particularly in the Far East where Oriental and Ayurvedic techniques were developed. These techniques involve pressure and are still widely used. The vigorous Swedish massage was developed in the 1800s by Per Henrik Ling, a gymnast. Modern Western massage is generally less vigorous than Swedish massage and focuses more on relaxation, well-being and points of muscle tension (Vickers & Zollman 1999).

Aromatherapy has also been widely used for centuries in many cultures, including Egypt and China. Rene Gattfesse and other French chemists developed modern aromatherapy in France in the 1900s (Young 2005). Gattfesse accidentally burned his hand in a perfume laboratory, then discovered that the burn healed after he applied

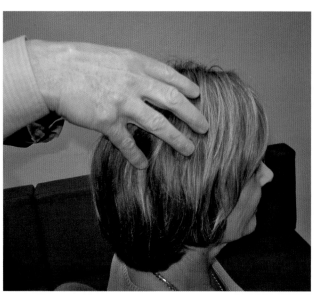

Fig. 49 **Head massage.** (Photograph courtesy of University of Edinburgh.)

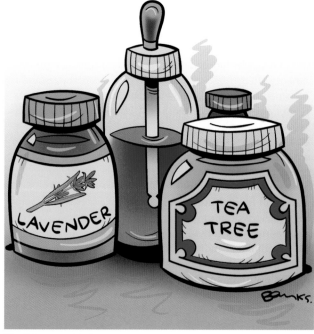

Fig. 50 **Essential oils.**

lavender oil to it. Modern aromatherapy is extremely popular and is widely used by the public through the form of aromatherapy candles and room vaporisers or diffusers. Many aromatherapy remedies are available over the counter in pharmacies.

Present regulation

There is no overall regulatory body that oversees aromatherapy or the massage therapies. There are about 12 organisations that govern aromatherapy and 9 that represent the massage therapies. Umbrella organisations include the Aromatherapy Organisations Council, the British Complementary Medicine Association and the Institute for Complementary Medicine. These bodies list approved practitioners and courses. A large variety of courses are offered up to diploma level in both massage and aromatherapy.

Role within conventional medicine

Both aromatherapy and massage are often used in conventional healthcare settings. Many nurses, midwives and allied healthcare professionals are trained in the use of these therapies, often within areas such as palliative care, mental health, pain management and paediatrics. Therapeutic sports massage is widely used by physiotherapists and offered by most sports medicine clinics. Massage can be found within a diverse range of healthcare settings from chronic pain clinics, hospices, labour wards to intensive care units.

Many general practices now offer access to some massage therapies.

A typical patient would be one who suffers from long-term anxiety and neck pain. If the GP feels that the pain is related to tension, the patient may be referred to one of the practice nurses who has trained in aromatherapy for a trial of massage therapy. The consultation takes around 90 minutes. A large amount of emphasis is placed on a peaceful atmosphere, with soft music and a specially designed massage couch. Various essential oils are used throughout the massage with greatest attention being placed on areas of increased muscle tension in the neck. The massage promotes a feeling of general well-being, relaxation and reduced muscle tension. The treatment will be carried out at monthly intervals if the patient feels she has benefited from the session.

Baby massage

Baby massage has become extremely widely used, particularly in neonatal units and intensive care environments. Baby massage is a technique that aims to promote well-being and to introduce the baby, even preterm infants, to the comfort of physical touch. Midwives often perform massage and teach the techniques to the infant's mother. More and more mothers use baby massage themselves to develop bonding with their infants and to promote relaxation of both mother and baby. Using warm hands and a non-toxic oil like olive oil, gentle strokes are applied to the baby, particularly to the chest, abdomen and limbs. These sessions are often continued until the baby starts to crawl. They are commonly used for babies with special needs, particularly those involving sensory and cognitive deprivation.

Table 26	**Other uses of essential oils**
Oil	**Use**
Tea tree oil	Athlete's foot, cold sores, head lice (topical)
Eucalyptus oil	Colds, sinusitis (inhaled)
Lavender oil	Burns, bites, cuts (topical)
Geranium	Acne (topical)
Peppermint	Asthma, colic, headache (inhaled)

Applications of oils

There are over 100 essential oils in therapeutic use and they have many roles other than as an adjunct to massage (Table 26). Essential oils used in aromatherapy can be added to massage oil to be used topically in therapeutic massage. They can also be inhaled from vaporisers or diffusers, candles, applied topically, added to baths or ingested. It is thought that their smell stimulates olfactory receptors, triggering the limbic system and promoting an emotional response.

Ling thought that massage therapies enhanced the circulation of lymph, but more important may be their enhancement of relaxation and anxiety reduction. The hand movements are used to reduce tension and stiffness. Part of this effect may be due to endorphin release. Many different massage techniques are available and some common ones are described in Table 27.

Evidence of efficacy

Some trials have shown limited benefits from massage and aromatherapy but studies are often of poor methodological quality with small patient numbers. Most trials of aromatherapy or massage have looked at short-term psychological outcomes rather than long-term symptomatic relief. There is little good quality evidence to support aromatherapy and the massage therapies.

Furlan and colleagues (2002) conducted a systematic review for the Cochrane Library of massage for low back pain. They appraised eight randomised controlled trials and suggested that massage might be beneficial, especially when combined with exercises and education.

Fellows and colleagues (2004) also generated a Cochrane systematic review of the role of aromatherapy and massage for symptom relief in patients with cancer. They showed short-term benefits on psychological well-being. Nevertheless, a subsequent randomised controlled trial by Soden and colleagues (2004) of aromatherapy massage in a hospice setting that looked at longer-term benefits showed no improvement in pain control, anxiety or quality of life.

Hanley and colleagues (2003) conducted a randomised controlled trial of therapeutic massage in the management

Table 27	**Examples of different massage therapies**
Swedish massage involves vigorous and deep massage techniques	
Aromatherapy massage utilises gentler techniques and essential oils added to massage oil	
Deep tissue and sports massage uses deep finger pressure to release muscle tension	
Manual lymph drainage uses techniques to expel toxins through stimulating lymph circulation	
Shiatsu is a Japanese technique that stimulates key pressure points through acupressure	
Ayurveda or Indian techniques again stimulate key pressure points particularly of the head	

of stress. They showed that despite very strong patient preference for massage it had no advantage over relaxation tapes used for stress relief.

Smith and colleagues (2004) conducted a Cochrane systematic review of complementary and alternative therapies for pain management in labour. One randomised controlled trial of aromatherapy was reviewed which showed no benefit.

There is limited evidence of efficacy supporting infant massage. Vickers and colleagues (2004) conducted a systematic review for the Cochrane Database. In it they reported that there is little evidence to show that massage for preterm infants is of benefit for developmental outcomes. Ohgi et al (2004) reported a randomised controlled trial of swaddling versus massage in the management of excessive crying in infants with cerebral injuries. They found that swaddling was a more effective intervention than massage in this group.

Safety issues

There is little evidence of sustained benefit from aromatherapy and the massage therapies, yet there is also little evidence of significant adverse events. Essential oils should never be ingested unless under the direct instructions of a qualified aromatherapist and discussion with the patient's doctor. The essential oils used for aromatherapy can be highly toxic if ingested undiluted and there have been case reports of serious toxicity in toddlers who have inadvertently ingested these oils. These toxic effects have included cases of hepatocellular necrosis and disseminated intravascular coagulation.

Massage should be avoided over infected skin and in conditions like deep venous thrombosis. It should not generally be used in early pregnancy or cases of malignancy without prior consultation with a doctor.

STOP THINK
- Despite the lack of good quality evidence for the use of massage therapies and aromatherapies many patients may find them beneficial and they are relatively risk-free.

Key points

- Few risks from these treatments.
- A child who ingests essential oils should be referred to hospital immediately.
- Due to the lack of formal regulation it is important that doctors advise patients to check that practitioners have recognised credible qualifications.

Sources of further information

- British Complementary Medicine Association: http://www.bcma.co.uk
- Essential oil toxicity from TOXBASE, National poisons information service: http://www.spib.axl.co.uk
- General information on massage and aromatherapy: http://www.channel4.com/health/microsites/C/comp_medicine/index.html
  http://www.bbc.co.uk/health/complementary
- Institute for Complementary Medicine: http://www.i-c-m.org.uk
- Resources on aromatherapy from the US: http://www.aromaweb.com

Reflexology

Janet Skinner

What is reflexology?

Reflexology involves the application of pressure and massage by the fingers and thumbs to specific reflex areas particularly of the feet, but also the hands and ears.

History and background

The origins of reflexology date back to ancient times when early Egyptian wall paintings showed examples of hand and foot massage. In the early 20th century, an ENT surgeon called William Fitzgerald noticed that pressure on one part of the body caused effects in others (Young 2005). The concepts of zones of the body running vertically from the head to the toes was developed and 'zone therapy' began (Vickers &

Zollman 1999). Maps were created showing the reflections of the body onto the soles of the feet. Modern reflexology was developed in the 1930s when a physiotherapist called Eunice Ingham systematically charted the entire body onto the feet.

Reflexologists believe that energy flows through the body in zones. There are ten zones that run throughout the body depicting organs and systems, and all of them are reflected onto the feet and hands. It is thought that stimulating these zones of the hands and feet, as shown in Figure 51, can have beneficial effects on the distant areas of the body that they represent. Reflexology charts are pictures of the soles of the feet with the rest of the body mapped out on them. Reflexologists believe that tenderness or 'grittiness' in these specific areas indicate disease in the mapped organ and that they can diagnose and treat disease by palpating the feet.

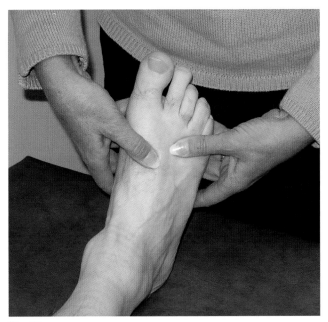

Fig. 51 **Reflexology massage.**

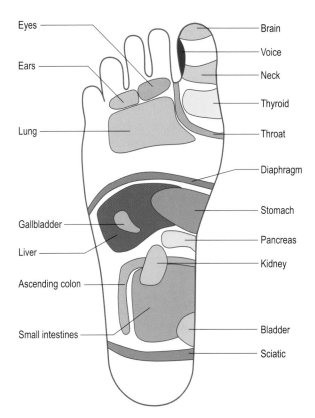

Fig. 52 **Example of a reflexology chart.**

Regulation

Reflexology has no overarching obligatory regulatory structure. Many people have called for voluntary self-regulation of reflexology and the Forum for Reflexology was created in 1999 to monitor and set standards. It also contains a list of qualified regulated practitioners.

Uses of reflexology

Early reflexologists divided the body up into ten vertical reflex zones with five being represented on each foot. These zones are said to link energy paths and that reflexology restores the 'balance' of these energy systems that flow through the body regaining 'equilibrium'. The left side of the body is represented on the left foot and vice versa.

Reflexologists believe that the build-up of waste products can be felt in the soles of the feet. They can detect these areas which highlight problems elsewhere in the zone. They press on and 'crush' these areas, reportedly leading to removal of waste products from distant organs. Reflexology is normally used in chronic conditions such as asthma, back pain, functional bowel disorders, headaches and stress. An example of a simplified reflexology chart with some of the right-sided organs mapped onto the feet is shown in Figure 52.

Vacuflex reflexology uses pads and vacuum boots to stimulate the reflex points. Metamorphic reflexology uses circular movements of the hands and feet.

Role in conventional medicine

Reflexology is less widely used within conventional medicine than many of the other complementary and alternative therapies. While some nurses and allied healthcare professionals are trained in reflexology it is less widely offered as a service, both within general practices and hospital medicine. It is less well integrated than similar therapies such as massage and aromatherapy and is infrequently offered as an NHS service.

Evidence and efficacy issues

There is very little good quality evidence to support the efficacy of reflexology. Few randomised controlled trials exist and those that do are generally of poor methodological quality. There are no Cochrane Collaboration systematic reviews that specifically address the therapeutic role of reflexology. One single blind trial of reflexology for irritable bowel syndrome exists in which reflexology was of no benefit in terms of the experience of pain, altered bowel habit, or abdominal distension in 35 patients who were randomised to receive either standard or reflexology foot massage (Tovey 2002).

Ross and colleagues (2002) carried out a pilot study to evaluate the effect of reflexology on mood and symptom rating of advanced cancer patients. Patients ($n=26$) were again randomised to conventional or reflexology foot massage. Both therapies were pleasurable to patients but there were no significant effects from either on mood or other common symptoms.

Brygge and colleagues (2001) performed a controlled trial of reflexology for people with asthma. Twenty patients received either real or simulated reflexology for 10 weeks. Objective lung function did not improve but subjective measures such as quality of life and need for medication improved in both groups. They concluded that reflexology had no specific effect on asthma apart from the placebo effect.

Williamson and colleagues (2002) conducted a randomised controlled trial of reflexology for menopausal symptoms. In it 76 women were randomised to real or simulated reflexology over nine sessions. Mean anxiety and depression scores fell in both the reflexology and the control groups, again suggesting the importance of the placebo effect and the role of therapeutic touch.

White and colleagues (2000) reported a blinded investigation looking at the accuracy of reflexology charts in diagnosis. Eighteen patients with one of six different medical conditions were examined by blinded reflexologists. There was poor inter-rater reliability between examiners and they were also poor at determining whether a condition was present or not. There is little or no other evidence to support the diagnostic ability of either reflexology charts or reflexologists themselves.

Currently there is insufficient evidence to advocate reflexology and there is a clear need for further good quality clinical studies.

Safety issues

Reflexology is relatively free of risk of adverse events but again should not be carried out in early pregnancy or in people with chronic medical conditions without consultation with their doctor first. It has been suggested that it may interfere with drug metabolism, particularly that of insulin. It should not be performed if medical conditions of the foot are present, for example gout, osteoarthritis or peripheral vascular disease.

Sources of further information

- Association of Reflexologists: http://www.aor.org.uk
- British Reflexology Association: http://www.britreflex.co.uk
- General information on reflexology: http://www.bbc.co.uk/health/complementary/therapies_reflex.shtml http://www.channel4.com/health/microsites/C/comp_medicine/reflexology.html
- Reflexology forum: http://www.reflexologyforum.org/

Case study

Irritable bowel syndrome

A young female patient has long-term problems with bloating and abdominal discomfort. It is felt that the symptoms are related to irritable bowel disease. She has failed to respond to standard therapy and makes an appointment to see a local private reflexologist on the recommendation of a friend.

Sessions involve the examination of the feet looking for hard areas that may indicate a build-up of toxins. These reflex points are massaged to sweep away waste from the bowel aiming to relieve symptoms. It is said that symptoms may initially become worse as toxins are released. Several sessions will be carried out over the next few weeks.

- In the BMJ's Minerva in 2002 it was reported that in a private health clinic in London for one hour it cost £20 to consult with a doctor or £40 to consult with a reflexologist.

Key points

- The evidence base to support the efficacy of reflexology as a therapeutic or diagnostic intervention is, to date, lacking.
- There is no evidence for adverse effects, other than the potential for delayed or mis-diagnosis.
- There is not, as yet, a single professional regulatory body for reflexology.

Nutritional therapy

Margaret R. Ritchie

Awareness of the role of nutrition in the prevention and treatment of disease is not a new concept. As early as 400 BC, Hippocrates (460–370 BC) was noted as stating 'let food be your medicine and medicine be your food'.

Food contains a variety of chemicals such as proteins, carbohydrates including complex carbohydrates such as fructoligosaccharides, fats and fatty acids, macronutrients, micronutrients, vitamins, minerals and bioactive components including phytochemicals. Phytochemicals are non-nutritive components in the plant-based diet ('phyto' is from the Greek word meaning plant) that possess substantial anti-carcinogenic (cancer preventing) and anti-mutagenic (anti-DNA damaging) properties (Surh 2003). Table 28 lists some facts supported by nutritional therapy.

Table 28 **Facts supported by nutritional therapy**

- Evidence from clinical and laboratory studies links nutritional factors and cancer risk.
- A single serving of vegetables contains more than 100 different phytochemicals (Surh 2003).
- Over 1000 different phytochemicals have demonstrated cancer-preventive properties.
- 400 potential plant compounds are currently under investigation in phase I, phase II and phase III trials (Surh 2003).
- In addition to phytochemicals, plants contain at least 12 000 natural chemicals produced for structural, hormonal, attractant and chemoprotective purposes (Mazur & Adlercreutz 1998, 2000).
- The use of plant biochemicals and vitamins as a therapy relies on the medicinal properties and actions of a number of these compounds.
- Up to 80% of cancers of the breast, bowel and prostate may be preventable by diet (Cummings & Bingham 1998).

What is nutritional therapy?

Nutritional therapy is the use of a special diet to balance the body and to prevent illness. A nutritional therapist will advise people how to improve their overall health by a careful study of what their body really needs in terms of food, vitamins and minerals based on careful analysis of an individual's general state of health, diet and lifestyle.

Philosophy of nutritional therapy

The use of nutrition, nutritional therapy and functional foods in disease management and prevention is based on a general philosophy that dietary manipulation or supplementation that includes specific nutrients will enable healing or prevent disease. A macrobiotic diet is based on the Chinese philosophy of yin and yang. Yin and yang foods can be adjusted by a nutritional therapist to restore the body to heath.

Nutritional therapy uses diet in the prevention and treatment of illness and to restore the body to a natural, healthy equilibrium. Subclinical deficiencies in nutrients, non-nutrients, vitamins and minerals (deficiencies which are too slight to result in obvious diseases such as scurvy or anaemia, but which are enough to affect the body's ability to function efficiently) are responsible for disease and weakness in the body. The symptoms of such a deficiency may include fatigue, susceptibility to colds, skin ailments and lethargy. Longer-term deficiencies are reported to contribute to obesity, heart disease, cancer, digestive disorders, premature ageing and death. Nutritional therapists believe that the Western (unhealthy) diet causes overfeeding but undernourishment due to the lack of food with adequate nutritional value. A healthy diet is one in which the food eaten provides all the essential nutrients for the body.

Poor health is also attributable to food allergies or intolerances and such foods should be avoided, while other foods, which have therapeutic properties, should be included in the diet.

What is good nutrition?

Nutritional therapists believe that the main ingredients of good nutrition and supplementation are:

- vitamins and minerals (Table 29)
- amino acids
- lipids and derivatives

- herbs
- others including acidophilus, bioflavonoids, yeast, co-enzyme Q10, enzymes, charcoal, bee and flower pollen, royal jelly, seaweeds and derivatives, and spirulina and chlorella.

Basic nutritional diagnoses

There are three basic diagnoses made by a nutritional therapist:

- allergy (or intolerance) to food
- nutritional deficiencies (often subclinical)
- toxic overload.

What happens in a nutritional therapy consultation?

A consultation (Fig. 53) usually lasts for one hour, during which time the nutritional therapist will:

1. Take a full case history including:
   - assessment of full diet history including eating habits, alcohol intake and smoking
   - identification of lifestyle issues such as exercise patterns, emotional and physical history
   - taking note of current and previous medication
   - taking note of physical symptoms and any additional symptoms.

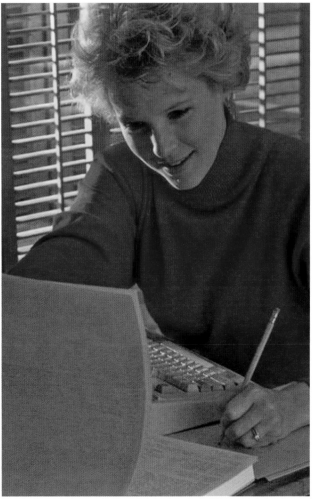

Fig. 53 **Nutritional therapist at work.** (Photograph courtesy of University of St. Andrews.)

Table 29 **Vitamins and minerals**	
Vitamins	**Minerals**
■ Vitamin A (retinol, carotene)	■ Calcium
■ B1 thiamine, B2 riboflavin, B3 niacin, B5 pantothenic acid, and B6 pyridoxine, B12 cobalamin, cyanocobalamin, folic acid and biotin	■ Chlorine
	■ Chromium
	■ Copper
■ Vitamin C (ascorbic acid)	■ Iodine
■ Vitamin D (calciferol, viosterol)	■ Iron
■ Vitamin E (tocopherol)	■ Magnesium
■ Vitamin F (fatty acids), vitamin H (biotin)	■ Molybdenum
■ Vitamin K (menadione)	■ Potassium
■ Vitamin M (folic acid), vitamin P (bioflavonoids)	■ Selenium
■ Vitamins T and U	■ Sulphur
	■ Vanadium
	■ Zinc

2. Conduct various nutritional therapy assessment tests such as
   - hair analysis for trace minerals
   - urine and blood analysis to measure glucose intolerance, vitamins, insulin, thyroid function
   - sweat analysis
   - muscle testing
   - use of a questionnaire to assess specific nutrient intake.
3. Assess dietary intake of vitamins and minerals (Fig. 54).
4. Recommend appropriate treatment tailored for each individual that may include:
   - dietary alteration to increase intake of specific nutrients
   - nutritional supplementation based on identification of dietary deficiencies
   - inclusion of specific foods to counteract the effect of food allergies which have been identified.

Role within conventional medicine

Nutritional therapy has been shown to help in a number of conditions such as high blood pressure (Most 2004), fatigue (Tamizi & Tamizi 2002, Vazquez 1998), constipation and other digestive disorders (Friedman 1989), rheumatism and arthritis (Soeken 2004), healing and recuperation following surgery or injury (Collins 2003, Fearon & Luff 2003), skin problems (Marino & King 1980), psychological and behavioural problems (Koo 1984, Bellisle 2004), neuralgia and inflammation (Ho et al 2004), osteoporosis (Heer et al 2004), pregnancy (Bitler & Currie 2005), postnatal illness (Walker & Wilging 2000), stress and viruses (Fields-Gardner & Fergusson 2004) and cancer (Jatoi et al 2005).

Contraindications – potential nutrient–drug interactions

Some foods may interact with conventional drugs and as such, the therapist and patient should be aware of current drug therapy and foods that may be contraindicated.

- Liquorice may interact with blood pressure lowering drugs, corticosteroids (prednisolone), diuretics (furosemide or thiazide) or cardiac drugs such as digoxin.
- Fruit juice and colas may interfere with some antibiotics.

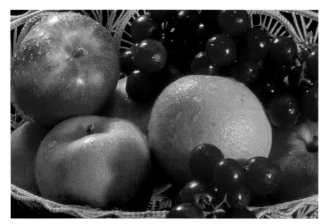

Fig. 54 **Vitamin- and mineral-containing foods.**

Case study

Background
Mr X presented with excessively sweaty, clammy hands from which he had suffered for 20 years. He suffered from regular chest infections and had a long-term sinus problem. He complained of low energy and colic, especially in the lower bowel. He reported feeling very stressed as a result of being a managing director of two companies.

Investigations
- Blood pressure (diastolic) was slightly high (93 mmHg)
- Alcohol intake high (30–40 units per week)
- Diet high in animal fats (ham and beef) and refined foods (pasta and bread)
- Organ function tested using Chapman reflex points (method for assessing organ function via specific points on the body, follows similar points to acupuncture).

Recommendations
- Silymarin (liver herb)
- Vitamin and mineral formula including several herbs such as basil, *Achyranthes* root, dog wood, *Ginkgo biloba*, and the amino acid tyrosine
- Reduce intake of alcohol and refined foods
- Increase intake of omega-3 fatty acids, foods with low glycaemic index, vegetables.

Results
Six weeks later sleep pattern improved, no bowel pain, energy levels increased (now at gym twice a week), sinus problems reduced, hands much less sweaty.

STOP THINK
- Some foods may interact with drug therapies
- Which patients would benefit from nutritional therapy?
- Can other lifestyle factors (such as increasing exercise, stress reduction, stopping smoking, increased relaxation) be changed during a course of nutritional therapy?

- Grapefruit and grapefruit juices enhance the absorption of ciclosporin used in organ transplantation, and may lead to increased toxicity.
- Dairy or milk products should not be taken with tetracycline antibiotics, or laxatives such as Dacodyl, Duco-lax and Fleet
- broccoli and brussel sprouts (rich in vitamin K) may diminish the anticoagulant property of blood thinners such as warfarin.
- Watercress may interfere with metabolism of paracetamol.
- Garlic may affect the enzyme CYP2E1.
- Foods rich in tyramine such as broad bean pods (fava beans), pickled herring, Chianti, aged cheeses such as Stilton and Roquefort, should not be taken with monoamine oxidase inhibitors (MAOIs). Foods rich in tyramine may also interact with isoniazid, used for tuberculosis.
- Tuna and mackerel should also be avoided during isoniazid therapy.

References

Adler S R, Fosket J R 1999 Disclosing complementary and alternative medicine use in the medical encounter: a qualitative study in women with breast cancer. Journal of Family Practice 48(6):453–458

Adlercreutz H, Mazur W 1997 Phyto-oestrogens and Western diseases. Annals of Medicine 29(2):95–120

Ang-Lee M K, Moss J, Yuan C S 2001 Herbal medicines and perioperative care. Journal of the American Medical Association 286(2):208–216

Arendt-Nielsen L, Nielsen J C, Bjerring P 1991 Double-blind, placebo controlled comparison of paracetamol and paracetamol plus codeine – a quantitative evaluation by laser induced pain. European Journal of Clinical Pharmacology 40(3):241–247

Asser S M, Swan R 1998 Child fatalities from religion-motivated medical neglect. Pediatrics 101(4):625–629

Baker L, Wagner T H, Singer S et al 2003 Use of the internet and e-mail for health care information: results from a national survey. Journal of the American Medical Association 289(18):2400–2406

Barnes J, Anderson LA, Phillipson JD 1996 Herbal medicines, 2nd edn. Pharmaceutical Press, Bath.

Barnes J, Mills S Y, Abbot N C 1998 Different standards for reporting ADRs to herbal remedies and conventional OTC remedies. British Journal of Clinical Pharmacology 45(5):496–500

Barnes P M, Powell-Griner E, McFann K et al 2004 Complementary and alternative medicine use among adults: United States, 2002. Advance data from vital and health statistics No. 343. Online. Available: http://www.cdc.gov/nchs/data/ad/ad343.pdf 1 June 2005

Barrett B, Marcband L, Scheder J et al 2004 What complementary and alternative medicine practitioners say about health and health care. Annals of Family Medicine 2(3):253–259

Barrett S 2003 Some thoughts about faith healing. Quackwatch. Online. Available: http://www.quackwatch.org/01QuackeryRelatedTopics/faith.html 1 June 2005

Barrios A 2001 A theory of hypnosis based on principles of conditioning and inhibition. Contemporary Hypnosis 18(4):163–203

BBC 1999 Britons turning to alternative cures. BBC News 23 August. Online. Available: http://news.bbc.co.uk/2/hi/health/426432.stm 1 June 2005

Beecher H K 1955 The powerful placebo. Journal of the American Medical Association 159:1602–1606

Bellisle F 2004 Effects of diet on behaviour and cognition in children. British Journal of Nutrition 92(suppl 2):S227–S232

Belon P, Cumps J, Ennis M et al 2004 Histamine dilutions modulate basophil activation. Inflammation Research 53(5):181–188

Berman B M 2001 Complementary medicine and medical education. BMJ 322(7279):121–122

Berman B 2005 Cochrane complementary medicine field. About the Cochrane Collaboration, Issue 2. Online. Available: http://www.mrw.interscience.wiley.com/cochrane/clabout/articles/COMPMED/frame.html 7 June 2005

Bernardi L, Sleight P, Bandinelli G et al 2001 Effect of rosary prayer and yoga mantras on autonomic cardiovascular rhythms: comparative study. BMJ 323:1446–1449

Bible 1984 The Holy Bible: New International Version. Hodder & Stoughton, London

Bitler M P, Currie J 2005 Does WIC work? The effects of WIC on pregnancy and birth outcomes. Journal of Policy Analysis and Management 24(1):73–91

BMA & RPSGB (British Medical Association and Royal Pharmaceutical Society of Great Britain) 2005 British national formulary (BNF) 50. BMA Publishing, London (produced bi-annually). Online. Available: http://www.bnf.org

Boon H, Brown J B, Gavin A, Westlake K 2003a Men with prostate cancer: making decisions about complementary/alternative medicine. Medical Decision Making 23:471–479

Boon H, Westlake K, Stewart M et al 2003b Use of complementary/alternative medicine by men diagnosed with prostate cancer: prevalence and characteristics. Urology 62:849–853

Boyd H 1989 Introduction to homoeopathic medicine, 2nd edn. Beaconsfield Publishers, Beaconsfield

Brauer R B, Stangl M, Stewart J R et al 2003 Acute liver failure after administration of herbal tranquilizer kava-kava (Piper methysticum). Journal of Clinical Psychiatry 64(2):216–218

Brigo B, Serpelloni G 1991 Homeopathic treatment of migraines: a randomised double-blind controlled study of sixty cases (homeopathic remedy versus placebo). Berlin Journal on Research in Homoeopathy 1(2):98–106

British Medical Association 1993 Complementary medicine: new approaches to good practice. Oxford University Press, Oxford

British Medical Association Board of Science and Education 2000 Acupuncture: efficacy, safety and practice. Harwood, Amsterdam

British Medical Association General Practitioners Committee 1999 Referrals to complementary therapists: guidance for GPs. British Medical Association, London

Brygge T, Heinig J H, Collins P et al 2001 Reflexology and bronchial asthma. Respiratory Medicine 95(3):173–179

Burton B 2003 Complementary medicines industry in crisis after recall of 1546 products. BMJ 326(7397):1001

Byrd RC 1988 Positive therapeutic effects of intercessory prayer in a coronary care unit population. Southern Medical Journal 81(7):826–829

Calabrese E J, Baldwin L A 1998 Hormesis as a biological hypothesis. Environmental Health Perspectives 106(suppl 1):357–362

Cancer Research UK 2002 Cancer Research UK Charity Number 1089464. Online. Available: http://www.cancerhelp.org.uk/help/default.asp?page=2657

Caspi O, Bell I R, Rychener D et al 2000 The tower of Babel: communication and medicine: an essay on medical education and complementary-alternative medicine. Archives of Internal Medicine 160(21):3193–3195

Chenoy R, Hussain S, Tayob Y et al 1994 Effect of oral gamolenic acid from evening primrose oil on menopausal flushing. BMJ 308:501–503

Clinical Standards Advisory Group 1994 Back pain. HMSO, London

Cochrane Collaboration 2005 The Cochrane Library Issue 1, 2005. John Wiley & Sons. Online. Available at http://www.cochrane.org

Collins N 2003 Protein-energy malnutrition and involuntary weight loss: nutritional and pharmacological strategies to enhance wound healing. Expert Opinion on Pharmacotherapy 4(7):1121–1140

Cooke G 2003 Crafted prayer: the joy of always getting your prayers answered. Sovereign World, Tonbridge, Kent

Council Directive 2002/46/EC of 10 June 2002 on the approximation of the laws of member states relating to food supplements. OJ L183/51 2002; 12 July

Cucherat M, Haugh M C, Gooch M et al 2000 Evidence of clinical efficacy of homeopathy. A meta-analysis of clinical trials. European Journal of Clinical Pharmacology 56(1):27–33

Cummings J H, Bingham S A 1998 Diet and the prevention of cancer. BMJ 317:1636–1640

Department of Health (UK) 2004 Regulation of herbal medicine and acupuncture: proposals for statutory regulation. Department of Health. Online. Available: http://www.dh.gov.uk/assetRoot/04/08/35/09/04083509.pdf 1 June 2005

Dickens P, Tai Y T, But P P et al 1994 Fatal accidental aconitine poisoning following ingestion of Chinese herbal medicine: a report of two cases. Forensic Science International 67(1):55–58

Dobson R 2003 Half of general practices offer patients complementary medicine. BMJ 327(7426):1250

Dossey L 1993 Healing words: the power of prayer and the practice of medicine. Harper, San Francisco

Dossey L 2004 The dark side of consciousness and the therapeutic relationship. Excerpts from an address to the Sixth Annual Alternative Therapies Symposium and Exhibition, San Diego, 2002. In: Schlitz M, Amorok T, Micozzi M Consciousness and healing integral approaches to mind–body medicine. Churchill Livingstone, Philadelphia, PA. DVD Audio. Transcript available: http://www.noetic.org/research/ch_book/files/Dossy.pdf 1 June 2005

EBM Working Group 1992 Evidence-based medicine: a new approach to teaching the practice of medicine. Journal of the American Medical Association 268(17):2420–2425

Eisenberg D M, Kessler R C, Foster C et al 1993 Unconventional medicine in the United States. Prevalence, costs and patterns of use. New England Journal of Medicine 382(4):246–252

Eisenberg D M, Davis R B, Ettner S L et al 1998 Trends in alternative medicine use in the United States, 1990–1997: results of a follow-up national survey. Journal of the American Medical Association 280(18):1569–1575

Eisenberger N I, Lieberman M D 2004 Why rejection hurts: a common neural alarm system for physical and social pain. Trends in Cognitive Sciences 8(7):294–300

EMEA 2005 European Medicines Agency website. Online. Available: http://www.emea.eu.int 17 June 2005

Ernst E 2000 The role of complementary and alternative medicine. BMJ 321(7269):1133–1135

Ernst E 2003 Chiropractic spinal manipulation for back pain. British Journal of Sports Medicine 37(3):195–196

Ernst M, Lee M H 1985 Sympathetic vasomotor changes induced by manual and electrical acupuncture of the Hoku point visualized by thermography. Pain 21(1):25–33

Ernst E, Pittler M H 1999 Ginkgo biloba for dementia: a systematic review of double-blind, placebo-controlled trials. Clinical Drug Investigation 17(4):301–308

Ernst E, White A 1997 Acupuncture: safety first. BMJ 314(7091):1362

Ernst E, White A (eds) 1999 Acupuncture: a scientific appraisal. Butterworth-Heinemann, Oxford

Ernst E, White A 2000 The BBC survey of complementary medicine use in the UK. Complementary Therapies in Medicine 8(1):32–36

Eskinazi D 1999 Homeopathy re-visited: is homeopathy compatible with biomedical observations? Archives of Internal Medicine 159(17):1981–1987

Expert Group on Vitamins and Minerals 2003 Safe upper levels for vitamins and minerals. Food Standards Agency, UK

Fearon K C, Luff R 2003 The nutritional management of surgical patients: enhanced recovery after surgery. Proceedings of the Nutrition Society 62(4):807–811

Fellows D, Barnes K, Wilkinson S 2004 Aromatherapy and massage for symptom relief in patients with cancer. The Cochrane Database of Systematic Reviews, Issue 3

Fields-Gardner C, Fergusson P, American Dietetic Association et al 2004 Nutrition intervention in the care of persons with human immunodeficiency virus infection: position of the American Dietetic Association and Dietitians of Canada. Canadian Journal of Dietetic Practice and Research 65(3):132–135

Fink M, Gutenbrunner C, Rollnik J et al 2001 Credibility of a newly designed placebo needle for clinical trials in acupuncture research. Forschende Komplementärmedizin und Klassische Naturheilkunde 8(6):368–372

Food Labelling Regulations 1996 (as amended). The Stationery Office, London

Frenkel M A, Borkan J M 2003 An approach for integrating complementary-alternative medicine into primary care. Family Practice 20(3):324–332

Friedman G 1989 Nutritional therapy of irritable bowel syndrome. Gastroenterology Clinics of North America 18(3):513–524

Fugh-Berman A 2000 Herb–drug interactions. Lancet 355(9198):134–138

Furlan A D, Brosseau L, Imamura M et al 2002 Massage for low-back pain. The Cochrane Database of Systematic Reviews, Issue 2

Garrison D W, Foreman R D 1994 Decreased activity of spontaneous and noxiously evoked dorsal horn cells during transcutaneous electrical nerve stimulation (TENS). Pain 58(3):309–315

Gatrad A R, Sadiq R, Sheikh A 2003 Multifaith chaplaincy. Lancet 362:748

George J, Ioannides-Demos L L, Santamaria N M et al 2004 Use of complementary and alternative medicines by patients with chronic obstructive pulmonary disease. Medical Journal of Australia 181(5):248–251

Giveon S M, Liberman N, Klang S et al 2004 Are people who use 'natural drugs' aware of their potentially harmful side effects and reporting to family physician? Patient Education and Counselling 53(1):5–11

GMC 1998 Seeking patients' consent: the ethical considerations. General Medical Council. Online. Available: http://www.gmc-uk.org/standards/consent.htm 1 June 2005

GMC 2000 Report of the visit to University of Edinburgh Faculty of Medicine 25–26 October 2000. Online. Available: http://www.gmc-uk.org/med_ed/visits/edinburgh.rtf 7 June 2005

GMC 2001 Good medical practice. General Medical Council. Online. Available: http://www.gmc-uk.org/standards/GMP.pdf 1 June 2005

GMC 2002 Tomorrow's doctors: recommendations on undergraduate medical education. General Medical Council. Online. Available: http://www.gmc-uk.org/med_ed/tomdoc.pdf 1 June 2005

Gray J A M 1997 Evidence-based healthcare: how to make health policy and management decisions. Churchill Livingstone, Edinburgh

Green M 1998 After Alpha. Kingsway, Eastbourne

Greenhalgh T 1999 Narrative based medicine: narrative based medicine in an evidence based world. BMJ 318(7179):323–325

Gruzelier J 1998 A working model of the neurophysiology of hypnosis: a review of the evidence. Contemporary Hypnosis 15(1):3–21

Guo H F, Tian J, Wang X et al 1996 Brain substrates activated by electroacupuncture of different frequencies (I): comparative study on the expression of oncogene c-fos and genes coding for three opioid peptides. Molecular Brain Research 43(1–2):157–166

Han J S, Sun S L 1990 Differential release of enkephalin and dynorphin by low and high frequencies electroacupuncture in the central nervous system. Acupuncture the Scientific International Journal 1(1):19–27

Han J S, Terenius L 1982 Neurochemical basis of acupuncture analgesia. Annual Review of Pharmacology and Toxicology 22:193–220

Han J S, Chen X H, Sun S L et al 1991 Effect of low- and high-frequency TENS on Met-enkephalin-Arg-Phe and dynorphin A immunoreactivity in human lumbar CSF. Pain 47(3):295–298

Hanley J, Stirling P, Brown C 2003 Randomised controlled trial of therapeutic massage in the management of stress. British Journal of General Practice 53(486):20–25

Harlow T, Greaves C, White A et al 2004 Randomised controlled trial of magnetic bracelets for relieving pain in osteoarthritis of the hip and knee. BMJ 329(7480):1450–1454

Harris P, Rees R 2000 The prevalence of complementary and alternative use among the general population: a systematic review of the literature. Complementary Therapies in Medicine 8(2):88–96

Harris W S, Gowda M, Kolb J W et al 1999 A randomized, controlled trial of the effects of remote, intercessory prayer on outcomes in patients admitted to the coronary care unit. Archives of Internal Medicine 159(19):2273–2278

Hawton K, Simkin S, Deeks J et al 2004 UK legislation on analgesic packs: before and after study of long term effect on poisonings. BMJ 329(7474):1076–1080

Hay D, Hunt K 2000 Understanding the spirituality of people who don't go to church: a report on the findings of the adults' spirituality project at the University of Nottingham. University of Nottingham, Nottingham

Heer M, Mika C, Grzella I et al 2004 Bone turnover during inpatient nutritional therapy and outpatient follow-up in patients with anorexia nervosa compared with that in healthy control subjects. American Journal of Clinical Nutrition 80(3):774–781

Hesketh T, Zhu W X 1997 Traditional Chinese medicine: one country, two systems. BMJ 315(7100):115–117

Ho E, Boileau T W, Bray T M 2004 Dietary influences on endocrine-inflammatory interactions in prostate cancer development. Archives of Biochemistry and Biophysics 428(1):109–117

House of Lords Select Committee on Science and Technology 2000 Complementary and alternative medicine, Sixth Report. TSO, London. Online. Available: http://www.publications.parliament.uk/pa/ld199900/ldselect/ldsctech/123/12301.htm 1 June 2005

Howell F 2004 Ireland's workplaces, going smoke free. BMJ 328(7444):847–848

Huang W F, Wen K C, Hsiao M L 1997 Adulteration by synthetic therapeutic substances of traditional Chinese medicines in Taiwan. Journal of Clinical Pharmacology 37:344–350

Hypericum Depression Trial Study Group 2002 Effect of Hypericum perforatum (St John's wort) in major depressive disorder: a randomized, controlled trial. Journal of the American Medical Association 287(14):1807–1814

Jatoi A, Williams B A, Marks R et al 2005 Exploring vitamin and mineral supplementation and purported clinical effects in patients with small cell lung cancer: results from the Mayo Clinic lung cancer cohort. Nutrition and Cancer 51(1):7–12

Kane M 2004 Research made easy in complementary and alternative medicine. Churchill Livingstone, Edinburgh

Kaye A D, Clarke R C, Sabar R et al 2000 Herbal medicines: current trends in anaesthesiology practice – a hospital survey. Journal of Clinical Anaesthesia 12(6):468–471

Kessler R C, Davis R B, Foster D F et al 2001 Long-term trends in the use of complementary and alternative medical therapies in the United States. Annals of Internal Medicine 135(4):262–268

King D E, Bushwick B 1994 Beliefs and attitudes of hospital inpatients about faith healing and prayer. Journal of Family Practice 39(4):349–352

Kirsch I, Sapirstein G 1998 Listening to Prozac but hearing placebo: a meta-analysis of antidepressant medication. Prevention and Treatment 1(1 June)

Ko R J 1998 Adulterants in Asian patent medicines. New England Journal of Medicine 339(12):847

Koenig H G 2000 Religion, spirituality and medicine: application to clinical practice. Journal of the American Medical Association 284(13):1708

Koenig H G 2004 Taking a spiritual history. Journal of the American Medical Association 291(23):2881

Koo L C 1984 The use of food to treat and prevent disease in Chinese culture. Social Science and Medicine 18(9):757–766

Kreitzer M J, Mitten D, Harris I et al 2002 Attitudes toward CAM among medical, nursing, and pharmacy faculty and students: a comparative analysis. Alternative Therapies in Health and Medicine 8(6):44–47, 50–53

Le Bars P L, Katz M M, Berman N et al 1997 A placebo-controlled, double-blind, randomized trial of an extract of Ginkgo biloba for dementia. Journal of the American Medical Association 278(16):1327–1332

Lee A, Done M L 1999 The use of nonpharmacologic techniques to prevent postoperative nausea and vomiting: a meta-analysis. Anesthesia and Analgesia 88(6):1362–1369

Leibovici L 2001 Effects of remote, retroactive intercessory prayer on outcomes in patients with bloodstream infection: randomised controlled trial. BMJ 323(7327):1450–1451

Lewit K 1991 Manipulative therapy in rehabilitation of the locomotor system, 2nd edn. Butterworth Heinemann, Oxford

Lewith G T, Johal W B, Walach H (eds) 2002 Clinical research in complementary therapies. Churchill Livingstone, Edinburgh

Liberti L E, Der Marderosian A 1978 Evaluation of commercial ginseng products. Journal of Pharmaceutical Sciences 67(10):1487–1489

Linde K, Ramirez G, Mulrow C D et al 1996 St John's wort for depression – an overview and meta-analysis of randomized clinical trials. BMJ 313(7052):253–258

Linde K, Clausius N, Ramirez G et al 1997 Are the clinical effects of homoeopathy placebo effects? A meta-analysis of placebo-controlled trials. Lancet 350(9081):834–843

Lipman L, Dale J, MacPherson H 2003 Attitudes of GPs towards the provision of acupuncture on the NHS. Complementary Therapy Medicine 11(2):110–114

Lo B, Quill T, Tulsky J 1999 Discussing palliative care with patients. Annals of Internal Medicine 130(9):744–749

Lo B, Ruston D, Kates L W et al 2002 Discussing religious and spiritual issues at the end of life: a practical guide for physicians. Journal of the American Medical Association 287(19):749–754

Loudon I (ed) 1997 Western medicine: an illustrated history. Oxford University Press, Oxford

Lundeberg T 1999 Acupuncture in headache. Cephalagia 19 suppl. 25:65–68

Ma K W 1992 The roots and development of Chinese acupuncture: from prehistory to early 20th century. Acupuncture in Medicine 10(suppl):92–99

McCaffrey A M, Eisenberg D M, Legedza A T R et al 2004 Prayer for health concerns: results of a national survey on prevalence and patterns of use. Archives of internal Medicine 164(8):858–862

Mackenzie G, Parkinson M, Lakhani A et al 1999 Issues that affect patient/physician discussion of complementary therapies. Patient Education and Counselling 38(2):155–159

MacPherson H, Thomas K, Walters S et al 2001 The York acupuncture safety study: a prospective survey of 34,000 treatments by traditional acupuncturists. BMJ 323(7311):486–487

Manheimer E, White A, Berman B et al 2005 Meta-analysis: acupuncture for low back pain. Annals of Internal Medicine 142(8):651–663

Marino D D, King J C 1980 Nutritional concerns during adolescence. Pediatric Clinics of North America 27(1):125–139

Martyn C 1995 Measuring the unmeasurable. BMJ 310(6990):1338

Mason S, Tovey T, Long A F 2002 Evaluating complementary medicine: methodological challenges of randomised controlled trials. BMJ 325(7368):832–834

Mathie R T 2003 The research evidence base for homeopathy: a fresh assessment of the literature. Homeopathy 92(2):84–91

Matthews D A, McCullough M E, Larson D B et al 1998 Religious commitment and health status: a review of the research and implications for family medicine. Archives of Family Medicine 7(2):118–124

Mazur W, Adlercreutz H 1998 Natural and anthropogenic environmental oestrogens: the scientific basis for risk assessment. Naturally occurring oestrogens in food. Pure and Applied Chemistry 70(9):1759–1776

Mazur W, Adlercreutz H 2000 Overview of naturally occurring endocrine – active substances in the human diet in relation to human health. Nutrition 16:654–687

Meade T W, Dyer S, Browne W et al 1995 Randomised comparison of chiropractic and hospital outpatient management for low back pain: results from extended follow up. BMJ 311(7001):349–351

Medicines Control Agency 2002 Safety of herbal medicinal products. Online. Available: http://medicines.mhra.gov.uk/ourwork/licensingmeds/herbalmeds/HerbalsSafetyReportJuly2002_Final.pdf 1 June 2005

Melchart D, Linde K, Fischer P et al 1999 Echinacea for preventing and treating the common cold. The Cochrane Database of Systematic Reviews, Issue 1

Melchart D, Linde K, Fischer P et al 2005 Acupuncture for idiopathic headache (Cochrane Review). The Cochrane Library Issue 2 John Wiley & Sons, Chichester

MHRA 2005a Medicines and Healthcare Products Regulatory Agency website. Online. Available: http://www.mhra.gov.uk 1 June 2005

MHRA 2005b Yellowcard website. Online. Available: http://www.yellowcard.gov.uk 1 June 2005

Miller L G 1998 Herbal medicinals: selected clinical considerations focusing on known or potential drug–herbal interactions. Archives of Internal Medicine 158(20):2200–2211

Mills S 1988 Alternatives in healing: an open-minded approach to finding the best treatment for your health problems. Grange Books, London

Mills S Y 2001a The House of Lords report on complementary medicine: a summary. Complementary Therapies in Medicine 9(1):34–39

Mills S 2001b Regulation in complementary and alternative medicine. BMJ 322:158–160

Mills S, Budd S 2000 Professional organisation of complementary and alternative medicine in the United Kingdom 2000: a second report to the Department of Health. Centre for Complementary Health Studies, University of Exeter, Exeter

Minerva 2002 BMJ 325:606

Ministry of Health, New Zealand 2003 Director General's privileged statement under section 98 of the Medicines Act 1981. Online. Available: http://www.moh.govt.nz/moh.nsf/0/0de600666a1711a8cc256cc f0064d574 1 June 2005

Monroe M H, Bynum D, Susi B et al 2003 Primary care physician preferences regarding spiritual behaviour in medical practice. Archives of Internal Medicine 163(22):2751–2756

Most M M 2004 Estimated phytochemical content of the Dietary Approaches to Stop Hypertension (DASH) diet is higher than in the control study diet. Journal of the American Dietetic Association 104(11):1725–1727

Murray S A, Kendall M, Boyd K et al 2004 Exploring the spiritual needs of people dying of lung cancer or heart failure: a prospective qualitative interview study of patients and their carers. Palliative Medicine 18(1):39–45

Muscari-Tomaioli G, Allegri F, Miali E et al 2001 Observational study of quality of life in patients with headache receiving homeopathic treatment. British Homoeopathic Journal 90(4):189–197

Myers D G 1999 Is prayer clinically effective? Reformed Review 53(2):93–102

National Population Health Studies 1994/1998 Perspectives on complementary and alternative health care: a collection of papers prepared for Health Canada 2001, Online. Available: http://www.hc-sc.gc.ca/hppb/healthcare/pubs/comp_alt/index.html June 2005

NCCAM 2004 The use of complementary and alternative medicine in the United States. National Center for Complementary and Alternative Medicine. Online. Available: http://nccam.nih.gov/news/camsurvey_fs1.htm 7 June 2005

NCCAM 2005 National Center for Complementary and Alternative Medicine website. Online. Available: http://www.nccam.nih.gov 1 June 2005

Neal R 2001 Report by David M. Eisenberg, MD, on educational issues pertaining to complementary and alternative medicine in the United States. Journal of Alternative and Complementary Medicine 7(suppl 1):41–43

Neighbour R 2004 The inner consultation: how to develop an effective and intuitive consulting style, 2nd edn. Radcliffe Medical Press, Abingdon

NeLH 2005 Hitting the headlines. UK National Health Service Electronic Library for Health. Online. Available: http://www.nelh.nhs.uk/hth/archive2.asp 10 June 2005

Newman Dorland W A (ed) 2000 Dorland's illustrated medical dictionary, 29th edn. Saunders, London

Ng T H, Chan Y W, Yu Y L et al 1991 Encephalopathy and neuropathy following ingestion of a Chinese herbal broth containing podophyllin. Journal of the Neurological Sciences 101(1):107–113

Nitzan U, Lichtenberg P 2004 Questionnaire survey on use of placebo. BMJ 329(7472):944–946

Novey D W 2000 Clinician's complete reference to complementary and alternative medicine. Mosby, St Louis

Ohgi S, Akiyama T, Arisawa K et al 2004 Randomised controlled trial of swaddling versus massage in the management of excessive crying in infants with cerebral injuries. Archives of Disease in Childhood 89(3):212–216

Owen D, Lewith G T 2001 Complementary and alternative medicine in the undergraduate medical curriculum: the Southampton experience. Medical Education 35(1):73–77

Owen D K, Lewith G, Stephens C R 2001 Can doctors respond to patients' increasing interest in complementary and alternative medicine? BMJ 322(7279):154–158

Pascoe GmbH 2002 Expertenkreis Naturmedizin: Naturmedizin Ausbildungssituation an Deutschen Hochschulen. Online. Available: http://www.expertenkreisnaturmedizin.de 17 June 2005

Paterson C, Dieppe P 2005 Characteristic and incidental (placebo) effects in complex interventions such as acupuncture. BMJ 330(7501):1202–1205

Pickar J G 2002 Neurophysiological effects of spinal manipulation. Spine Journal 2(5):357–371

Pietroni P 1991 The greening of medicine. Gollancz, London

Pittler M H, Ernst E 2000 Ginkgo biloba extract for the treatment of intermittent claudication: a meta-analysis of randomized trials. American Journal of Medicine 108(4):276–281

Porter R 1988 Before the fringe: 'Quackery' and the eighteenth-century medical market. In: Cooter R (ed) Studies in the history of alternative medicine. Macmillan, London, p 1–27

Radin D I, Nelson R D 1989 Evidence for consciousness-related anomalies in random physical systems. Foundations of Physics 19(12):1499–1514

Rainville P, Hofbauer R, Paus T et al 1999 Cerebral mechanisms of hypnotic induction and suggestion. Journal of Cognitive Neuroscience 11(1):110–125

Rao J K, Mihaliak K, Kroenke K et al 1999 Use of complementary therapies for arthritis among patients of rheumatologists. Annals of Internal Medicine 131(6):409–416

Rees L, Weil A 2001 Integrated medicine. BMJ 322(7279):119–120

Resch K, Hill, S, Ernst E 1997 Use of complementary therapies by individuals with arthritis. Clinical Rheumatology 16:371–375

Roberts L, Ahmed I, Hall S 2000 Intercessory prayer for the alleviation of ill health. The Cochrane Database of Systematic Reviews, Issue 2

Rosner F 1999 Can an amulet cure leukaemia? Journal of the American Medical Association 282:307

Ross C S, Hamilton J, Macrae G et al 2002 A pilot study to evaluate the effect of reflexology on mood and symptom rating of advanced cancer patients. Palliative Medicine 16(6):544–545

Roth L U, Maret-Maric A, Adler R H et al 1997 Acupuncture points have subjective (needling sensation) and objective (serum cortisol increase) specificity. Acupuncture in Medicine 15(1):2–5

Rowin J, Lewis S L 1996 Spontaneous bilateral subdural hematomas associated with chronic *Ginkgo biloba* ingestion. Neurology 46(6):1775–1776

Sackett D L, Straus S E, Richardson W S et al 2000 Evidence-based medicine: how to practice and teach EBM, 2nd edn. Churchill Livingstone, New York

Saks M 1996 From quackery to complementary medicine: the shifting boundaries between orthodox and unorthodox medical knowledge. In: Cant S, Sharma U (eds) Complementary and alternative medicines: knowledge in practice. Free Association Books, London, p 27–43

Samanta A, Samanta J 2003 Legal standard of care: a shift from the traditional Bolam test. Clinical Medicine 5:443–446

Satterlund M J, McCaul K D, Sandgren A K 2003 Information gathering over time by breast cancer patients. Journal of Medical Internet Research 5(3):e15. Online. Available: http://www.jmir.org/2003/3/e15/15 June 2005

SCHIN 2002 Prodigy: evidence based clinical guidance. Sowerby Centre for Health Informatics at Newcastle, Newcastle

Schmidt K, Ernst E 2004 Assessing websites on complementary and alternative medicine for cancer. Annals of Oncology 15(5):733–742

Schmidt K, Pittler M H, Ernst E 2001 Bias in alternative medicine is still rife but is diminishing. BMJ 323(7320):1071

Schmidt K, Jacobs P A, Barton A 2002 Cross-cultural differences in GPs' attitudes towards complementary and alternative medicine: a survey comparing regions of the UK and Germany. Complementary Therapies in Medicine 10(3):141–147

Schofield P E, Juraskova I, Butow P N 2003 How oncologists discuss complementary therapy use with their patients: an audiotape audit. Support Care Cancer 11(6):348–355

Sheikh A 1997 Quiet room is needed in hospitals for prayer and reflection. BMJ 315:1625

Sheldon T 2004 Netherlands to crack down on complementary medicine. BMJ 328:485

Shibuya K, Ciecierski C, Guindon E et al 2003 WHO framework convention on tobacco control: development of an evidence based global public health treaty. BMJ 327(7407):154–157

SIGN-BTS (Scottish Intercollegiate Guidelines Network, British Thoracic Society) 2004 Guideline 63: British guideline on the management of asthma. Scottish Intercollegiate Guidelines Network, Edinburgh

Simpson J A, Weiner E S C (eds) 1989 Prayer. Oxford English dictionary, 2nd edn. Clarendon Press, Oxford

Simpson W F 1989 Comparative longevity in a college cohort of Christian Scientists. Journal of the American Medical Association 262(12):1657–1658

Slifman N R, Obermeyer W R, Aloi B K et al 1998 Contamination of botanical dietary supplements by *Digitalis lanata*. New England Journal of Medicine 339(12):806–811

Sloan R P, Bagiella E, Powell T 1999 Religion, spirituality, and medicine. Lancet 353(9153):664–667

Smith C A, Collins C T, Cyna A M et al 2004 Complementary and alternative therapies for pain management in labour. The Cochrane Database of Systematic Reviews, Issue 2

Soden K, Vincent K, Craske S et al 2004 A randomized controlled trial of aromatherapy massage in a hospice setting. Palliative Medicine 18(2):87–92

Soeken K L 2004 Selected CAM therapies for arthritis-related pain: the evidence from systematic reviews. Clinical Journal of Pain 20(1):13–18

Spencer J W, Jacobs J J 1999 Complementary/alternative medicine: an evidence based approach. Mosby, St Louis

Stevinson C, Pittler M H, Ernst E 2000 Garlic for treating hypercholesterolemia. A meta-analysis of randomized clinical trials. Annals of Internal Medicine 133(6):420–429

Stevinson C, Honan W, Cooke B et al 2001 Neurological complications of cervical spine manipulation. Journal of the Royal Society of Medicine 94(3):107–110

Stone J, Matthews J 1996 Complementary medicine and the law. Oxford University Press, Oxford

Straumsheim P, Borchgrevink C, Mowinckel P et al 2000 Homeopathic treatment of migraine: a double blind, placebo controlled trial of 68 patients. British Homoeopathic Journal 89(1):4–7

Surh Y J 2003 Cancer chemoprevention with dietary phytochemicals. Nature Reviews. Cancer 3(10):768–780

Swayne J (ed) 2000 Churchill Livingstone's international dictionary of homeopathy. Churchill Livingstone, Edinburgh

Swenson R, Haldeman S 2003 Spinal manipulative therapy for low back pain. Journal of the American Academy of Orthopaedic Surgeons 11(4):228–237

Szegedi A, Kohnen R, Dienel A et al 2005 Acute treatment of moderate to severe depression with hypericum extract WS 5570 (St John's wort): randomised controlled double blind non-inferiority trial versus paroxetine. BMJ 330(7490):503–506

Tamizi far B, Tamizi B 2002 Treatment of chronic fatigue syndrome by dietary supplementation with omega-3 fatty acids – a good idea? Medical Hypotheses 58(3):249–250

Tang J L, Zhan S Y, Ernst E 1999 Review of randomised controlled trials of traditional Chinese medicine. BMJ 319(7203):160–161

Tasaki K, Maskarinec G, Shumay D M et al 2002 Communication between physicians and cancer patients about complementary and alternative medicine: exploring patients' perspectives. Psycho-Oncology 11(3):212–220

Tate P 2003 The doctor's communication handbook, 4th edn. Radcliffe Medical Press, Abingdon

Thomas K J, Nicoll J P, Coleman P 2001 Use and expenditure for complementary medicine in England: a population based survey. Complementary Therapies in Medicine 9(1):2–11

Tian J H, Xu W, Zhang W et al 1997 Involvement of endogenous orphanin FQ in electroacupuncture-induced analgesia. Neuroreport 8(2):497–500

Tovey P A 2002 A single-blind trial of reflexology for irritable bowel syndrome. British Journal of General Practice 52(474):19–23

UK BEAM Trial Team 2004a United Kingdom back pain exercise and manipulation (UK BEAM) randomised trial: effectiveness of physical treatments for back pain in primary care. BMJ 329(7479):1377

UK BEAM Trial Team 2004b United Kingdom back pain exercise and manipulation (UK BEAM) randomised trial: cost effectiveness of physical treatments for back pain in primary care. BMJ 329(7479):1381

Vale S 1998 Subarachnoid haemorrhage associated with *Ginkgo biloba*. Lancet 352(9121):36

Vandenbroucke J P 1997 Homeopathy trials: going nowhere. Lancet 350(9081):824

Vanherweghem J L 1998 Misuse of herbal remedies: the cause of an outbreak of terminal renal failure in Belgium (Chinese herbs nephropathy). Journal of Alternative and Complementary Medicines 4(1):9–13

Vanherweghem J L, Depierreux M, Tielemans C et al 1993 Rapidly progressive interstitial renal fibrosis in young women: association with slimming regimen including Chinese herbs. Lancet 341(8842):387–391

Vas J, Méndez C, Perea-Milla E et al 2004 Acupuncture as a complementary therapy to the pharmacological treatment of osteoarthritis of the knee: randomised controlled trial. BMJ 329(7476):1216–1220

Vazquez E 1998 Managing weight loss with nutritional supplements. Positively Aware 9(2):49

Vickers A 2000 Recent advances: complementary medicine. BMJ 321(7262):683–686

Vickers A, Zollman C 1999 ABC of complementary medicine: massage therapies. BMJ 319(7219):1254–1257

Vickers A, Ohlsson A, Lacy J B et al 2004 Massage for promoting growth and development of preterm and/or low birth-weight infants. The Cochrane Database of Systematic Reviews Issue 2

Vincent C 2001 The safety of acupuncture. BMJ 323(7311):467–468

Walach H, Haeusler W, Lowes T et al 1997 Classical homeopathic treatment of chronic headaches. Cephalalgia 17(2):119–126

Walach H, Jonas W B, Lewith G 2002 The role of outcomes research in evaluating complementary and alternative medicine. In: Lewith G, Jonas W B, Walach H (eds) Clinical research in complementary therapies: principles, problems and solutions. Churchill Livingstone, London, p 29–45

Walker L O, Wilging S 2000 Rediscovering the 'M' in 'MCH' maternal health promotion after childbirth. Journal of Obstetric, Gynecologic, and Neonatal Nursing 29(3):229–236

Wang K W, Han J S 1990 Accelerated synthesis and release of angiotensin II in the rat brain during electroacupuncture tolerance. Science in China (B) 33(6):686–693

Wei H, Chung-long Huang L, Kong J 1999 The substrate and properties of meridians: a review of modern research. Acupuncture Medicine 17(2):134–139

Weir M 2003 Obligations to advise of options for treatment: medical doctors and complementary and alternative medicine practitioners. Journal of Law and Medicine 10(3):296–307

Wetzel M S, Kaptchuk T J, Haramati A et al 2003 Complementary and alternative medical therapies: implications for medical education. Annals of Internal Medicine 138(3):191–196

White A R, Williamson J, Hart A et al 2000 A blinded investigation into the accuracy of reflexology charts. Complementary Therapies in Medicine 8(3):166–172

White A, Hayhoe S, Hart A et al 2001 Adverse events following acupuncture: prospective survey of 32,000 consultations with doctors and physiotherapists. BMJ 323(7311):485–486

Whitmarsh T E, Coleston-Shields D M, Steiner T J 1997 Double-blind randomized placebo-controlled study of homoeopathic prophylaxis of migraine. Cephalalgia 17(5):600–604

Williamson J, White A, Hart A et al 2002 Randomised trial of reflexology for menopausal symptoms. BJOG: an International Journal of Obstetrics and Gynaecology 109(9):1050–1055

Wilt T J, MacDonald R, Ishani A 1999 β-sitosterol for the treatment of benign prostatic hyperplasia: a systematic review. British Journal of Urology International 83(9):976–983

Woelk H 2000 Comparison of St John's wort and imipramine for treating depression: randomised controlled trial. BMJ 321(7260):536–539

Woodard C 1959 A doctor heals by faith. Hodder and Stoughton, London

World Health Organization 1998 The World Health Organization Quality of Life Assessment (WHOQOL): development and general psychometric properties. Social Science and Medicine 46(12):1569–1585

World Health Organization 2002 WHO Policy Perspectives on Medicines No. 2. Traditional medicine – growing needs and potential. World Health Organization, Geneva

World Health Organization 2003 Traditional medicine. Fact Sheet No 134. World Health Organization. Online. Available: http://www.who.int/mediacentre/factsheets/fs134/en/print.html 1 June 2005

Yardley L, Furhham A 1999 Attitudes of medical and nonmedical students toward orthodox and complementary therapies: is scientific evidence taken into account? Journal of Alternative and Complementary Medicine 5(3):293–295

Young J 2005 Reflexology. BBC. Online. Available: http://www.bbc.co.uk/health/healthy_living/complementary_medicine/therapies_reflexology.shtml 1 June 2005

Zhou Y, Sun Y H, Shen J M et al 1993 Increased release of immunoreactive CCK-8 by electroacupuncture and enhancement of electroacupuncture analgesia by CCK-B antagonist in rat spinal cord. Neuropeptides 24(3):139–144

Zollman C, Vickers A 1999a ABC of complementary medicine: complementary medicine in conventional practice. BMJ 319(7214):901–904

Zollman C, Vickers A 1999b ABC of complementary medicine: complementary medicine and the patient. BMJ 319(7223):1486–1489

Zollman C, Vickers A 1999c ABC of complementary medicine: complementary medicine and the doctor. BMJ 319(7224):1558–1561

Zollman C, Vickers A 1999d ABC of complementary medicine: what is complementary medicine? BMJ 319:693–696

Index